LOSE WEIGHT
AND GAIN LIFE

Indicates clearly the path to be followed if you would reduce your weight to normal and healthy proportions.

Also in this series
BEFORE AND AFTER BABY COMES
CIDER APPLE VINEGAR
HEART AILMENTS
HIGH BLOOD PRESSURE
HONEY: NATURAL FOOD AND HEALER
HOW TO KEEP YOUNG AFTER FORTY
IMPROVE YOUR SIGHT WITHOUT GLASSES
MASSAGE AT YOUR FINGERTIPS
NERVE TROUBLES
RAW JUICES FOR HEALTH
RHEUMATISM AND ARTHRITIS
SKIN TROUBLES
STOMACH ULCERS AND ACIDITY
VITAMINS EXPLAINED SIMPLY
WOMAN'S CHANGE OF LIFE

LOSE WEIGHT AND GAIN HEALTH

*Prepared and produced by the Editorial Committee of
Science of Life Books*

Revised and extended by
Leonard Mervyn B.Sc., Ph.D., F.R.S.C.

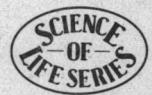

SCIENCE OF LIFE BOOKS
4-12 Tattersalls Lane, Melbourne, Victoria 3000

Seventh Edition, revised, enlarged and reset, 1984

© SCIENCE OF LIFE BOOKS 1984

Registered at the G.P.O. Sydney for transmission through the post as a book

This book is sold subject to the condition that it shall not, by way of trade or otherwise, be lent, re-sold, hired out, or otherwise circulated without the publisher's prior consent in any form of binding or cover other than that in which it is published and without a similar condition including this condition being imposed on the subsequent purchaser.

National Library of Australia card number
and ISBN 0-909911-03-07

Printed in Great Britain by
Richard Clay (The Chaucer Press) Ltd,
Bungay, Suffolk

Contents

		Page
	Foreword	7

Chapter

1.	The Dangers of Being Overweight	13
2.	The Healthy Weight	23
3.	The Reasons Why You are Overweight	31
4.	Feeding the Human Furnace	42
5.	Food Values and Fundamentals	59
6.	Vitamin and Mineral Needs when Reducing Weight	71
7.	The Experts' Views	82
8.	Weight Reducing Diet	102
	Index	111

Foreword

Overweight is one of the major health problems of the modern western world. It is a product of our affluent society. History shows that as standards of living rise so does the incidence of overweight. In Australia, for example, it has been estimated that eighteen per cent of girls and ten per cent of boys are overweight and that in the older age groups forty per cent of people are at least ten per cent overweight.

While overweight itself is not a disease it is closely associated with disorders such as gallstones, hypertension and diabetes and it can considerably add to the discomfort and pain of arthritis, rheumatism, gout, asthma and respiratory problems etc.

Overweight is often associated with chronic tiredness. More energy is required to move a heavier body, and all too often the effort is too great, so that overweight contributes to lack of exercise which in turn contributes further to the weight problem.

Stress is another contributory factor and many people under stress look for snacks or sweets to eat between meals. Eating becomes a way of escape from stress and of course this escape merely transforms a psychological problem into a physical problem.

Little needs to be said about the relationship of alcohol to obesity. Alcohol, like white sugar, provides an abundance of empty calories and nothing else. In Australia twenty-five per cent of all calories in the diet come from alcohol or sugar. The situation in the United States, where the populus is renowned for their sweet tooth, is probably worse, while in Britain and Europe the position is almost certainly no better than that in Australia. Little wonder forty per cent of the population in the older age groups are overweight.

Alcohol and sugar not only contribute directly to the weight problem but they have the effect of satisfying the appetite and reducing the intake of nutritious foods, thus lowering the standard of nutrition and paving the way for nutritional deficiencies.

Another villain in our western society is common salt. The average person eats far too much salt. Salt is included in many processed foods — cheese, canned foods, breakfast cereals, take-away foods, biscuits etc., are all salted to 'improve' their flavour. Our taste buds have been perverted by excessive amounts of salt since we were born. Salt interferes with the mineral and electrolyte balance in the body and an excess of salt causes fluid retention, which can contribute considerably to overweight. In order to function properly the body does need some salt, but only a small amount in comparison to what our food provides. Health authorities have recommended that our salt intake be limited to 5g (about ⅙ ounce) per day.

The way in which the body uses food varies from individual to individual. Some people find it hard to gain weight no matter what they eat, others seem to convert all foods into fat and, no matter how hard they try, they find it very difficult to lose weight. In both of these extreme circumstances medical advice should be sought as the problem may be only a symptom of some other more serious condition. A calorie-controlled, balanced diet combined with adequate exercise or active sport should be all that a healthy person needs to lose weight.

Here we must sound a warning about 'fad' diets — mono-diets and diets which do not provide a balanced intake of foods from the various food groups. Basically, our energy intake should be obtained as follows:

10–15 per cent of all calories from protein foods
55–60 per cent of all calories from carbohydrate foods and mainly from unprocessed foods (wholegrains etc.)
25–30 per cent of all calories from fats or oil

With these factors taken into consideration it must be remembered that diets providing less than 2,000 calories (8,200 kilojoules) per day are almost certain to provide insufficient vitamins and minerals to maintain a good standard of health, and therefore should not be adopted for more than a week or so unless vitamin and mineral supplements are used as a routine part of the daily programme. All too often the unfortunate overweight person reduces their calorie intake to a level which does not provide adequate amounts of vitamins and minerals and deficiency symptoms develop.

One of the groups most at risk from 'fad' diets are teenage girls. Growing children or adolescents should not attempt to follow any reducing diets unless under medical supervision.

Teenagers and growing children have a higher nutritional need than adults and a drastic reduction in their calorie intake may not only affect their growth and maturity but also pave the way for disorders such as anorexia nervosa, stomach upsets, anaemia, acne, skin problems etc.

'Fad' diets are those which fail to provide a balanced intake of food from the various food groups recognised by most nutritional Authorities throughout the world. These food groups may be summarized into the following categories:

1. Meat, eggs and fish
2. Milk, cheese and dairy products
3. Vegetables
4. Grains, flour, breakfast cereals
5. Fruit

Statistics clearly show a reduction in the lifespan with obesity even in a moderate ten to twenty per cent overweight. This can be readily appreciated when we realise that overweight is one of the causative factors in hypertension fifteen per cent of the Australian population suffer with high blood pressure) and that overweight is associated with the following disease states: adult-onset diabetes; hypercholesterolaemia; hypertriglyceridaemia;

hepatic disease; cholecystitus; female genital malignant disease; abdominal hernia; cerebovascular, accident and peripheral vascular disease.

The death rate due to hepatic disease, respiratory disease, arteriosclerotic heart disease, albuminuric acid and diabetes is increased by overweight. Clinical conditions made worse by overweight include angina pectoris, cardiac decompensation, respiratory disease, hiatus hernia and psychiatric conditions. Moreover, overweight can cause problems in clinical management involving anaethesia, surgical procedures and post-operative embolism.

It is little wonder then that life insurance companies consider the weight of an applicant when assessing life assurance premiums and where the risk is considered greater than normal appropriate loadings to premiums are introduced.

Overweight is in many cases a lifestyle problem and in its control our lifestyle may have to be modified or altered as part of our overall health programme. This is usually not difficult once the decision has been taken, and the following pages can assist you greatly with suggestions for making the necessary adjustments.

WILLIAM KING D.O., D.C.
New South Wales

1

The Dangers of Being Overweight

According to life insurance statistics, six out of ten people in this country at the age of forty are overweight. The same percentage of people — six out of ten — will be dangerously overweight by the time they reach the age of fifty. Approximately fifty per cent of them will not live to the age of sixty, and of the fifty per cent that do reach that age, the majority will be in very indifferent health, or chronically ill or organically diseased.

From the point of view of the life insurance companies, the fat or overweight person is a very bad risk indeed, and will only be accepted subject to 'special loading', that is, the payment of a high premium. As will be seen from life insurance graphs, the death rate increases sharply with every 2.5 kilos (five pounds) of weight we put on over the ideal weight. The ideal weight, by the way (according to the life insurance companies who have made a hundred years' study of this subject), is the weight of the average man or woman at the age of thirty.

Tables giving this ideal weight are on pages 28-29.

The Deadly Dangers of Being Overweight

Let us see what the medical profession says of excessive weight.

'All the world may love a fat man, but not for long — he doesn't live long,' was the stand taken by Dr Emerson V. Potter when, as chairman of a group of New York doctors, he addressed a joint legislative committee of New York State on problems of the ageing. He continued, 'Obesity is the greatest single hazard to human life in the nation today,' but he warned against strenuous dieting to bring down weight in a hurry — 'This is often more dangerous than obesity.'

Appealing for a publicity programme, urging more exercise and balanced diets, he said, 'Obesity curtails life, impairs vigour, increases fatigue, breaks down the liver, increases surgical risks, and is associated with hypertension, arteriosclerosis, and heart disease.'

Heart Diseases 50 per cent Higher

Here is an excerpt from a bulletin put out by the Metropolitan Life Insurance Company of the U.S.A:

'Overweights suffer more frequently and earlier from the major chronic conditions than do persons of normal weight. An example is hypertension, or high blood pressure, with heart disease.

'The death rate from coronary artery disease is fifty per cent greater among the overweight.

'Among those with twenty-five per cent excess body weight, the death rate from diabetes is eight times higher than among persons of normal weight.

'For every inch (2.5 cm) the waist measurement exceeds the chest measurement, the person may subtract two years from his life expectancy.'

Dr Louis I. Dublin and his associates at the Metropolitan Life Insurance Co. have shown that, of persons overweight up to fourteen per cent, the death rate from all causes is twenty-two per cent higher than among persons of normal weight. Among persons who are overweight from fifteen to twenty-four per cent, the death rate is forty-four per cent higher than among those of normal weight, and among persons who are overweight twenty-five per cent or more it is seventy-five per cent higher.

The Greatest Killer is Obesity

The evidence of thousands of medical records and case histories says that the overweight millions are the likeliest victims of heart disease, diabetes, liver disorders, artery hardening, and all the degenerative diseases of old age.

Dr Dublin has proved his point with cold figures. He selected 50,000 men and women insured by his company, whose only defect in the years 1925–1934 was obesity. In 1950 that group was compared with 50,000 persons who also had been in good health in 1925–1934 — but without obesity.

Dr Dublin found that for every two deaths in the normal weight group, three of the fat persons had died. Among overweight men, the death rate from heart disorders was fifty per cent higher than normal; among overweight women, seventy-five per cent, higher.

Diabetes was four times deadlier than in the normal weight group. The death rate from gallstones was twice the standard, and deaths from cirrhosis of the liver in men were more than two and a half times higher than normal. There was excess mortality from cancer of the liver and gall-bladder.

Dr Dublin also studied obese persons who reduced their weight to normal standards. The result: the death rate in men dropped one-fifth; in women, one-third.

As a country becomes increasingly wealthy its inhabitants are able to eat more and exercise less, so not surprisingly, the proportion of overweight people in that community rises steadily. For example, in the United States of America almost two-thirds of those over fifty years of age are at least ten per cent overweight. In Great Britain and the rest of Europe, less than one-quarter of the middle-aged citizens are overweight but unfortunately the proportion of overweight females is now approaching that of the United States. Australia, too, is nearer the American than the European situation.

There is no secret why there are 40 million 'fat' people in the U.S.A. — they eat too much. So says Dr Norman Schneeberg of the Einstein Medical Centre, Philadelphia, U.S.A. How is it that many people can maintain the same weight during the whole of their adult life, despite the fact that they eat huge quantities of food during this time? For example, studies amongst the Zulus of Africa who lead a natural life, eating natural food, have shown that their weight does not vary appreciably between 25 and 65 years of age after which it drops slightly. According to Dr Schneeberg it is due to the fact that the appetite, and therefore the amount of food consumed, is controlled by a tiny part of the brain he calls the 'appestat'. In most people who live a normally active life with no major stresses or strains the appestat works as efficiently in keeping their weight at the correct level, as does a thermostat in maintaining a constant temperature. What it does is to control the appetite by indicating when a person has had enough food. Too often food is eaten because it is there and not because it is needed. The appestat can only indicate to an individual that they have had enough, it can't stop them eating.

Strict dieting appears to alter the setting of the appestat in the same way in which we can reduce the temperature by reducing the setting of a thermostat. Similarly, of course, if our setting of the appestat is so high because of excessive eating, the appetite will be increased accordingly so that too much food intake will become the norm rather than the occasional exception. Once dieting has restored a healthier weight it should become no more difficult to maintain it with the appestat than it was at the old level. People often speak of prolonged dieting causing the stomach to contract and thus accept less food. This is not quite true, because what has really happened is that they have set their appestat lower so appetite is curtailed. Hence the only way to lose weight is to eat less and so maintain the appestat at the lower setting.

'The Plague of the Twentieth Century'

Dr Harry Johnson, Director of U.S.A. Life Extension Examiners, writes in *How to Live*:

'One of the more significant problems in nutrition is to impress on most people that their food requirements are less than their food consumption. Most people eat too much.

'Overweight might well be considered the plague

of the twentieth century. This is truly an insidious disease process which undermines the physical wellbeing and ultimately results in the degeneration and destruction of the body.

'This condition is not generally recognized as a serious menace to long life and activity.

'It is too often accepted with the expression that it is "natural" for this or that person to be fat.

'Overweight may be responsible directly and indirectly for more physical disability than any other disease.

'This fact is not generally recognized, because the ill-effects of overweight are insidious in their development, and when they become evident they manifest themselves in such a form as apparently not to be associated with their true cause.

'Very few laymen and not many physicians recognize, in overweight, potential diabetes, heart disease, kidney disease, gall-bladder disease, arterial hypertension, and innumerable other difficulties.

'The direct relationship between these is evident when we study the problem.

'Insurance company actuaries have definitely established the relationship between life expectancy and weight, and they find that with increasing weight there is a decreasing longevity.

'This excessive fat in the overweight person acts as a parasite, slowly sapping the energy and reserve of the organs of the body, and if allowed to continue for a long enough period will bring about its untimely destruction.'

Weight Consciousness

Dr Johnson continues: 'Very extensive and elaborate research work has been done to determine how much a person should eat each day.

'The exact calorific requirement for labouring men in different fields has been carefully studied.

'All of this is very interesting, but primarily of academic importance. For the average laymen practically no consideration need be given to calories. The important consideration is to watch the weight.

'If the weight increases above the normal, the intake of food is too great. If weight is being lost below the normal, the intake of food is inadequate.

'Every obese person should, without delay, become weight-conscious. He should make every effort to bring about a slow but constant loss — one or two pounds each week is sufficient.

'This is difficult and requires unusual perseverance and self-denial on the part of the patient. The "get-thin-quick" methods prescribed over the radio and in other advertisements are notoriously unsatisfactory and often hazardous.

'Their primary advantage lies in the economic return to the companies promoting them.

'Nature has provided all normal, healthy individuals with an appetite far in excess of what the body needs to carry on its daily work. There are various sensible diet routines which can satisfactorily bring about a gradual weight loss.

'No matter how limited the diet, it must always be balanced. Under these conditions the fat stored in the body will be utilized to make up the deficiency and a loss in weight will result.

Only One Safe Way to Reduce
'It is unwise to attempt to lose weight by indulging

in violent exercise. This is particularly true in the middle-aged and older person, as it may result in a serious strain on the heart and circulatory system.

'Any loss thus accomplished will usually be temporary. Moderate exercise is an essential part of any reducing programme, but it should be remembered that loss of weight is brought about by diet restriction and not by physical activity.

'There is no safe medication yet discovered which will bring about a loss in weight; there is no short-cut to this difficult assignment.

'But the reward of perseverance and close adherence to the diet restrictions is a longer, happier and much healthier life.

'A programme of weight reduction which has been found to be satisfactory with a great many patients includes moderate exercise with the diet restrictions.

'When the patient has been on this routine there has been no feeling of weakness, complaint of headache or other disturbing symptoms.

'After the first few weeks of diet restriction, the uncomfortable sensation of hunger has disappeared completely.

'The slow weight reduction serves a twofold purpose in that it tends to protect the patient from the harmful effects of too rapid loss and also assures the development of new habits of eating which will be easily adhered to for an indefinite period.'

It is a fallacy that middle-aged spread in women is due to the change of life. Studies have shown that the average weight of women rises steadily from thirty onwards without any sharp increase between the ages of forty-five and fifty-five when most women enter the menopause. It is usually at

THE DANGERS OF BEING OVERWEIGHT

middle-age that the increased weight becomes noticeable or troublesome.

We must therefore conclude that loss of excess weight is important not only from the point of view of appearance but because it can have a beneficial effect upon the health. Painful knees are extremely common in middle-aged and older women. Other joints, particularly the hips and ankles, may also be affected by excess weight in both men and women. The most important long term self-treatment for painful weight-bearing joints must therefore be a loss in weight.

When breathlessness is due to heat strain, high blood pressure or advancing years, it is usually eased by a reduction in weight. Another benefit is relief of chronic indigestion, which is often worse in an overweight person on lying down or bending forward. The indigestion is due to a partial escape of stomach contents upwards into the food pipe — a consequence much more likely in a fat individual.

Apart from these reliefs from existing conditions, there is no doubt that prevention of certain diseases can also occur by maintaining a lower body weight. Weight reduction can reduce the chances of a person developing diabetes or coronary thrombosis particularly for an individual who has relatives suffering from these complaints and who may have inherited similar tendencies. It is highly likely that weight reduction lessens the chances of developing gallstones. The 'five Fs' have been used to describe the person likely to suffer from this complaint, namely; female, fair, forty, fertile and fat. Only in the last factor does the individual have any control.

Women who are markedly overweight have more chance of developing complications when they are pregnant. There is also more risk of harm to the body as it develops. A feature of gross obesity in women is a lowered fertility rate due, in part, to infrequent menstruation in these people. Sometimes a decrease in weight will help a woman to conceive. Statistics show that overweight individuals have more accidents than those of more normal weight, perhaps due to a reduced agility. Major operations create greater hazards for the fat person because of the greater incisions required and the extra stress introduced into a body already prone to the greater strains induced by overweight.

2

The Healthy Weight

Dr Eugene Fisk, Medical Director, Life Extension Institute of New York writes:

'How many people, after they are thirty years of age, have a conformation of body that is in accord with proper ideals of health and symmetry?

'The average individual, as age progresses, gains weight until he reaches old age, when the weight usually decreases.

'This movement of weight is so universal that it has been accepted as normal, or physiological, whereas it is not normal, and is the result of disease-producing and life-shortening influences.

'Standards for weight and height at the various ages have been established by life assurance companies, but these standards, which show an increase in weight as age advances, by no means reflect standards of health and efficiency.

'They merely indicate the average condition of people accepted for life insurance.

'They demonstrate that, in the absence of pathology, the average weight for thirty years of age is the ideal weight to maintain throughout maturity. Experience shows that those so proportioned exhibit the most favourable mortality.

'After middle life, extreme light weight may not be incompatible with good health. A youthful figure, as a rule, reflects a superior vitality, other things being equal.

'The usual gain in weight is not an advantage but a handicap.'

'Slimming for the Million'

Dr Eustace Chesser, a Harley Street authority on the subject of obesity, writes, in *Slimming for the Million*:

'For years physicians and life insurance companies have studied the influence of body-weight upon health and life-span, and the tables which have been produced in consequence serve some useful purpose as a general standard of comparison.

'The very fact that such tables are deemed necessary by the insurance companies is a sufficiently clear indication that experience has taught them that overweight is a menace to health.

'It is safe to say that a person of normal weight has a much better chance of attaining a ripe old age than has one whose weight is excessive.

'Why do such companies increase their premium rates in the case of those overweight as judged by their tables?

'Certainly it is not a matter of mere prejudice, neither is it due to any lack of desire to do as much business as possible.

'The very large sums of money spent by such undertakings on advertising, the care and expense

THE HEALTHY WEIGHT

devoted to training their representatives, and the very keen competition for business which exists among them are plain indications that only one explanation answers these questions. In insurance parlance the obese are "bad lives".'

Three Physical Types

Dr Chesser continues:

'Take a good look at yourself! Weigh yourself up! For your shape and weight are very closely connected both with your bodily health and your outlook on life.

'In fact, one of the best guides to your health is your weight in relation to your shape and height.

'There are three main body types walking this earth, as you may have noticed if you have taken the trouble to observe:

1. Those who are slender, with a short body on long legs (small frame);
2. Medium-weight people with length of body and legs in good proportion (medium frame);
3. The 'heavily built', with a wide, long body on short legs (large frame).

'You can pick out these three groups quite easily at any swimming pool or bathing beach, for the world is made up of these three types. And your ideal weight depends, to some extent, upon which of these three classifications you belong to.

'That is why it is impossible to lay down hard-and-fast rules as to what is an ideal weight for people of any particular age or height.

'For example, most of the tables which indicate the weights regarded as ideal at various ages and heights allow a man of forty-four, 170cm, (5ft 7in) tall, an average weight of 68kg (150 pounds).

'But everything depends upon how that weight is distributed — in other words — upon the shape of the man . . .

The Ideal Weight
'The exact weight which can be regarded as ideal for a person about whom nothing is known beyond height and age, cannot be stated.

'It must be appreciated that such tables are compiled by striking an average from many thousands of persons, some more, some less, than average.

'But the bony framework in some is thicker and wider than in others, apart from structural differences. Five thousand perfectly healthy men will yield an average weight, yet this might not be the ideal weight for any one of them.

'Far better, then, for the guidance of the average reader, to provide a table showing the range within which a person should weigh.

'Other things being equal, they need not bother about their weight unless they find themselves outside these limits.

'Growth and development are usually complete in men at about twenty-five years, and in women at twenty years.

'Once the body has reached its normal, adult development, weight increase is almost invariably due to the accumulation of fat.

'A certain amount of fatty tissue is necessary, but all the fat which is favourable to health is usually acquired within five years of the completion of growth and development — that is, in men by the

THE HEALTHY WEIGHT

age of thirty, in women by twenty-five.

'The average man or woman, having reached these ages, has acquired the most favourable body-weight. Fortunate, indeed, are those who retain it!'

Weight tables giving average weights which are taken from countries of western civilisation include a large number of overweight people, so the average weight for older people is therefore not necessarily the normal or the best weight. For this reason, a better guide is to be found in the tables prepared by the New York Metropolitan Insurance Company. These take into account the ideal range of weights for people of small, medium and large builds and so allow for individual variation. They may be regarded as the best weights to be attained.

In the Height-Weight Tables that follow, the heights do not include footwear and weights given are exclusive of all clothing. Indoor female garments may be assumed to weigh 3kg (6 lbs); those of males are about 4.5kg (10 lbs).

WOMEN

Height		Small Frame		Medium Frame		Large Frame	
cm	ft. in.	kg	lb	kg	lb	kg	lb
150	4'11"	45-46	100-102	46.5-48.5	103-107	49-51	108-112
152	5'	47-48	104-106	48.5-50.5	107-111	51-53	112-116
155	5'1"	48-49	106-108	49.5-51	109-113	52-54	114-118
157	5'2"	49-50	108-110	50.5-52	111-115	53-54.5	116-120
160	5'3"	50-51	110-112	51-53	113-117	54-55.5	118-122
163	5'4"	51-52	112-114	52-54	115-119	54.5-56	120-124
165	5'5"	52-53	114-116	53-55	117-121	55.5-57	122-126
168	5'6"	53-54	116-118	54-56	119-123	56-58	124-128
170	5'7"	54-54.5	118-120	55-56.5	121-125	57-59	126-130
173	5'8"	54.5-55.5	120-122	56-57.5	123-127	58-60	128-132
175	5'9"	55.5-56	122-124	56.5-58.5	125-129	59-61	130-134
178	5'10"	56-57	124-126	57.5-60.5	127-133	61-63	134-138

MEN

Height		Small Frame		Medium Frame		Large Frame	
cm	ft.in.	kg	lb	kg	lb	kg	lb
160	5'3"	54-58	119-128	57.5-61.5	127-136	60.5-65.5	133-144
163	5'4"	55.5-59.5	122-131	59-63.5	130-140	62-67.5	137-149
165	5'5"	57-61.5	126-136	61-65.5	134-144	64-69.5	141-153
168	5'6"	58.5-63	129-139	62.5-66.5	137-147	66-71	145-157
170	5'7"	60.5-65	133-143	64-68.5	141-151	67.5-73.5	149-162
173	5'8"	61.5-66.5	136-147	66-70.5	145-156	69.5-75.5	153-166
175	5'9"	63.5-68.5	140-151	67.5-72.5	149-160	71-77	157-170
178	5'10"	65.5-70.5	144-155	69.5-74.5	153-164	73-79.5	161-175
180	5'11"	67-72	148-159	71-76	157-168	75-81.5	165-180
183	6'	69-74.5	152-164	73-78.5	161-173	76.5-84	169-185
185	6'1"	71-76.5	157-169	75.5-80.5	166-178	79-86	174-190
188	6'2"	73.5-79	162-174	78-82.5	167-182	85-89	187-196

Even without scales there are simple indications of the overweight condition. For example, if you can pick up thick rolls of fat between your fingers and thumbs at the following places: the back of the upper arm; below the shoulder blades; above and around the waist; and/or the hips, buttocks, tummy and upper thigh. Usually a few pounds of overweight are of no significance to the health, and it is only when an individual is ten per cent or more over his best weight (calculated from the tables) that there should be cause for concern. At this stage the presence of excess fat under the skin becomes obvious. In some men, however, fat is stored beneath the muscular layers of the abdomen. Hence, it is not obvious directly beneath the skin but there is still an increase in girth at the level of the navel. Here the only warning signs of excess weight will come from the scales.

3

The Reasons Why You are Overweight

A certain amount of fatty tissue is necessary because it acts as a heat-insulating layer beneath the skin. The vital organs, such as the kidneys, are also surrounded by fat which acts as a cushion against physical injury. Fat may be regarded as the main energy storage form and as such there must always be some present as an insurance against hunger and starvation.

According to Dr Eustace Chesser, growth and development are usually complete in men at about twenty-five years and in women at twenty years of age. So, once the body has reached its normal adult development, weight increase is almost invariably due to the accumulation of excess fat.

Before we consider the various reasons why we put on weight, we should dispose of one fallacy that is all too often put forward as an explanation of weight-gain. This is the idea that an upset in the glands can contribute to the laying-down of body fat. There is no doubt that a malfunctioning thyroid can upset the body's weight control but a weight increase is only one symptom amongst many and, on its own, it does not suggest the thyroid is involved. Over-production of stress hormones have also been popularly implicated in excessive weight increase but again the condition is rare and is invariably accompanied by other symptoms that can only be interpreted by a doctor. Hence, we may assume that in the vast majority of overweight people an upset in glandular metabolism is not a factor in their problem.

Heredity: Heredity may play a part since a tendency to overweight runs in many families. It has been observed that those who tend to put on weight have parents, grandparents, aunts, uncles, brothers and sisters with the same tendency to lay down fat. Of course, when families eat together regularly the chances are that the members all eat incorrectly or excessively. Despite this, however, it now looks as if most people who are overweight are born with a tendency to be that way.

Some evidence of this has come from the fact that adopted children usually take after their real parents in this respect and not after the families into which they are adopted. Similarly, studies of identical twins who have been separated at birth and brought up by different families indicate that their body weights stay almost identical. On the other hand, twins produced from two eggs (ie born at the same time but not identical) are further apart than identical twins and weight differences between them are far greater.

Modern research has discovered that people with an hereditary tendency to be overweight are, in fact, different from other people in the way they handle fat. Obese individuals, even during childhood, cannot dispose of fatty tissue as easily as others do. Once the fat is eventually broken down, these fat people cannot burn it up to produce the heat and energy so essential to maintaining a normal weight. In some way their method of metabolizing fat is different from normal individuals so they suffer accordingly.

An inherited liking for food by overweight people is another factor that leads to excessive weight. Observations on lean children have indicated that they have far more food dislikes than those children who tend to be fat. The desire for food in an obese person sometimes verges on addiction. In the words of one well-known American doctor: 'It seems to me that hunger in the obese might be so ravaging and voracious that we skinny physicians do not understand it.'

There is no doubt that these people with a tendency to put on weight easily are inclined to be less active than others, even before they put on weight, so this tendency is naturally increased as they grow heavier. It is possible that some individuals expend only half the amount of energy as others even when stationary. Less energy expenditure must inevitably lead to calories being laid down in the form of fat. The person who is always active and restless is rarely overweight. This inherent burning of calories explains why people of the same height and weight may differ dramatically in their dietary needs to maintain weight. The calorie intake of a fat person can be lower than that of a thin individual yet because of simple body expenditure of energy without exercise, that person will put on weight unlike his thin counterpart who literally 'burns' it away.

Lack of exercise: This represents the sole cause of excess weight in some people as they age, usually because they give up the active sports and exercise that they indulged in when younger. Too often also, advancing years and perhaps added responsibilities in one's job reduce the time available for exercise. Sometimes an active post becomes a sedentary one with a resulting decreased demand for energy expenditure. The process of becoming a car-owner of those who previously walked or cycled to work may be the factor contributing to weight gain. As energy expenditure decreases, the intake of food often stays the same or even increases so, unfortunately, lack of proportional decrease of food must inevitably lead to weight gain.

Do not underestimate the beneficial effects of increased exercise in reducing weight. An individual weighing 76 kg (168 pounds; 12 stones) would lose about one pound of weight whilst walking ten hours. This may at first might appear to be depressing to the weight watcher but there is another way of looking at it. What must be considered are the long term aspects of the problem. The same person, walking for an extra forty minutes per day, could lose 28g (1 ounce) of weight daily. Over a week this represents almost 200g (½ pound); at the end of a month nearly 1 kg (2 pounds) and more than 10 kg (20 pounds) in a year. On the other hand, an individual who used to walk for twenty minutes each to and from work, bus-stop or station who now drives to work is likely to gain that weight. Body weight gain is an insidious process.

Other examples of the relationship between exercise and food intake are numerous. A potato of medium size needs the energy expenditure involved in playing nine holes of golf to burn it away. A 50 g (2 ounce) bar of chocolate requires eighteen holes of golf. A glass of milk represents a walk of close on three miles. One lump of sugar equals a walk of one third of a mile. Even the mildest exercises add up in increasing energy expenditure and hence in reducing the tendency to lay down fat. Some important recent studies from the Department of Nutrition of the University of London have shown that exercise has the effect in people of normal weight of temporarily increasing the rate at which the body functions. This means that calories are burnt up at a faster rate when exercising an hour after a meal. The proof came by deliberately overfeeding thin people and finding that their weight did not increase as expected. Those who were overweight had lost this capacity to burn up extra food in this way and so weight gain resulted. However, once people had managed to lose weight this capacity to burn off extra calories was regained. Hence, once some weight has been lost, exercise can become doubly beneficial.

Social Factors

In the West, women, by their very way of life, are encouraged to overeat. There are pressures put on them to nibble at food as they prepare it. Often they regard themselves as human dustbins who will eat their children's left-overs rather than waste them. The family meal in the evenings of working days is an opportunity to partake of the main repast, which is usually a full-blown dinner which they also enjoy themselves. In the case of the working family, this may be in addition to a business lunch, where the combination of hospitality, restaurant meals and a more than usual intake of alcohol can cause an enormous increase in calories.

Most social gatherings involve eating and drinking alcoholic or other beverages, whether they are coffee mornings, charity lunches or dinner parties. No coffee morning is complete without biscuits, cake, confectionery and savories, all foods full of fat, sugar and calories. It is difficult for anyone to resist the temptation to have a second helping of a highly-fattening, delicious sweet that is overloaded with calories. The opportunities for extra-mural eating are more likely to fall to the stay-at-home mother and wife rather than to the working woman.

The housewife will find other, more psychological, pressures brought upon her to increase her desire to eat. Her life is often subject to the minor frustrations constant decisions and responsibilities in looking after the children. The boredom of daily household tasks can introduce lethargy and a mild depression which is often overcome by eating. Home entertainments, particularly television, because of their very inactivity induce a desire to eat. Even sophisticated advertisements for food can stimulate the taste-buds. Such temptations are not, of course, confined to the housewife, and the males of the household are just as likely to succumb to those extra, unnecessary calories.

The need to overeat that leads to difficulty in weight control occurs commonly in those people who have suffered a lack of affection during some period of their lives. They may be denied some of the major satisfactions of life and find solace in

THE REASONS WHY YOU ARE OVERWEIGHT 37

food. The problems in such people is in controlling the desire to eat. It takes a great deal of will-power to desist and, even if successful, the weight lost is usually regained within a short period when the original desire to eat asserts itself again. The ultimate situation is a series of ups and downs in body weight which is probably more harmful than a consistently maintained increase.

A recent study has indicated that the children who suffer most at school at the hands of other children are those who are fat. Ridicule of these youngsters is far greater than those of children with other afflictions. They are usually poor at games because of their condition. Other factors, however, lead to unhappiness in school children. They may come from broken homes, or were unwanted by their parents. This frequently results in gifts of sweets, chocolate and other confectionery by the parents as an attempt to make up for the affection they feel they are unable to give. Also, such gifts are too often rewards for effort or compensation for illness or hurt or simply a sop to the child's demands. Many very happy children have loving parents who will readily satisfy their children's demands for sweets, cakes, ice-cream and biscuits, often because the parents themselves, were when young, deprived of such luxuries.

Those who desire to have children and cannot will often eat to compensate for their disappointment. Simple everyday stress or tension, induced perhaps by a hated job or by an unhappy life, can lead to some people seeking solace in food. After all, eating and drinking are two of the basic pleasures of life and can, in some circumstances, compensate for lack of love and affection. The consequences, however, are dire, because these pleasures get out of proportion when they eventually become insufficient for the individual's need.

There are many people in this category who are content to remain overweight because they realize that they need to eat and the process becomes a reasonable compromise. There are others, though, who may feel unloved and unwanted and when they seek to overcome their loneliness in this way simply become fatter and less attractive and so become even more unhappy. Looking in the mirror they see themselves as undesirable persons whom nobody could possibly want to love. The net result is an even greater urge to eat, so the whole vicious circle starts again.

Hence the psychological state of an individual can often determine his or her desire to eat. In addition however, many modern psychologists believe that some people actually have an addiction to food in the same way as they may have one for alcohol, gambling or smoking. Of course, if the problem of overeating has its origin in any of these mental situations then professional advice is best sought. What we are more concerned with in this book is how an individual may lose weight safely and naturally when they are, or can be, in control of their own eating habits.

Despite the psychological and social pressures that assail us all, it is still a fact that some people, no matter what they eat, simply will not put on weight. It now looks as if biochemical differences in our body make-up can explain why some people are more prone to gaining weight than others. Apparently it may all depend upon the recently discovered 'brown fat' which is the powerhouse for turning food into heat. Thin people have more of it than those who are fat.

Some years ago a classic experiment was carried out by biochemist Sir Charles Dodds. He took a mixed batch of people and fed them double and treble their normal food intake. Those who were naturally slim did not put on an ounce but measurements of their metabolic rate indicated that this increased to burn up the extra calories. The rest of the group showed no change in metabolic rate and gained weight. This experiment has been repeated many times always with the same result.

If over-feeding does not necessarily produce weight gain neither will dieting lead to guaranteed weight loss. A recent study involved thirty women who were overweight and were put on a strict 1500 calories per day. After three weeks two of them actually gained weight; nine had failed to lose so much as an ounce and the rest had weight losses varying from a few ounces to five pounds.

There are other causes of weight gain. One has been described as 'carbohydrate hoarding'. Carbohydrates are the food constituents which make up starches, found in bread, cereals, grains, potatoes, root vegetables and nuts and sugars, richest in table sugar but also found in honey and fruits. Some people believe that a calorie from one type of food constituent (for example carbohydrate) is identical to that from any other type of constituent (say protein). However, according to Dr Richard Mackarness in his book *Eat Fat and Grow Slim*, carbohydrate hoarders have insufficient enzymes to convert carbohydrate to energy and so they make fat. These people should have a diet aimed at a high protein intake with low carbohydrate and normal fat levels. Carbohydrate hoarders should count carbohydrates and not calories. They must therefore find out what daily intake of carbohydrates suits them, by trial and error. Sugars should be avoided completely as should grains, bread and flour of all sorts. Some carbohydrate can be provided in fruits, nuts and starch-containing vegetables, but only in moderation. High protein foods such as meat, fish, eggs, cheese can be eaten in any quantity. Fibre can be provided by leafy vegetables.

Why Do You Want to Lose Weight?

This is a valid question to consider because it is important for the individual to know exactly why they wish to lose weight. It gives them an end result to aim for, which helps when the desire to reduce weight becomes less than that to eat. Once the lower weight is reached, however, there is a great sense of achievement which makes the problem of maintaining the lower weight that much easier to tackle. At the same time, if the end result of a weight loss brings the hoped-for benefits, that in itself is stimulus enough. The individual should, however, have some idea at the start of what those benefits will be.

One of the better incentives to lose weight is to relieve a physical condition that may have been exacerbated by the overweight condition. Ankles and knees represent the joints that take the brunt of the strain induced by excessive weight. Once middle-age has come and passed, the wear and tear of these joints is reflected in a very painful condition that usually starts on the inside of the knees. It is surprising how often a simple reduction in weight relieves the condition.

THE REASONS WHY YOU ARE OVERWEIGHT

There are cosmetic reasons for appearing slimmer. A young person may yearn for the fashionable clothes that seem to be confined to the slim. Increasing one's attractiveness to one's partner is often stimulus enough to lose weight. An impending holiday, where the person seeks a better figure to display on a beach, is one of the more common incentives to lose unsightly pounds.

There are those, of course, whose urge to eat dominates their lives and the only way they can achieve a weight reduction is to seek a fresh interest to take their minds off food. This may appear difficult or downright impossible for people such as housewives with young children to care for, but it can be done. Many young mothers help at school meal sessions where the sight of so much food, far from stimulating the appetite often suppresses it. Part-time jobs can increase the chances of alternative interests and in this way the urge to eat may be lessened. There are possibilities, for women in particular, to work at home because there is nothing better than being active to take the mind off food. Whether the activity is productive like knitting, secretarial work or model-making or is educational like attending evening classes, the facts show that those who follow these pursuits are less likely to develop the urge to eat than those who do nothing.

4

Feeding the Human Furnace

Dr Eustace Chesser, the authority on obesity, has this to say:

'Fat folk have a thin time these days! Quite apart from the prejudicial effect which excess weight has upon health, these are times in which lean men and slender woman are favoured. In all kinds of occupations, other things being equal, the lean are preferred to the fat.

'They look, and in fact are, more alert, fitter, better prepared for providing the quick results which are demanded of us today, both physically and mentally.

'The burden of excess fat cannot be laid down like a workman's tools at the end of the working day. It is here — a handicap — even through sleeping hours.

'Those who, whether through ignorance or love of good things, regularly over-eat, carry through life a heavier handicap than their excess pounds. The immortal Bard of Avon was among the first to draw attention to this when he said: "Fat paunches have lean pates; and dainty bits make rich the ribs, but bankrupt quite the wits."

'Various other references to the woes and deficiencies of the obese reveal clearly that Shakespeare recognized how heavy a burden the fat carry through life.

'The plain, unadulterated truth is that the overwhelming majority of fat people owe their condition to one sad fact: they eat too much, or at any rate eat too much of the fat-forming foods. Most people consume at least twice as much food as the body strictly requires.

'In these days, conscious that corpulence is not regarded as an attractive feature of her sex, modern Eve often takes great pains to keep her food consumption down lest she should put on weight.

Get a Sense of Food Values

'The object of fat in the human body is to provide a reserve of fuel. Unlike a reserve fund of money the more you have of this fuel reserve in the body does not make you better off, but exactly the reverse.

'It is stored very economically, since fat is the most concentrated of all fuels. In other words, a little goes a long way.

'Different kinds of food produce varying amounts of heat, and their relationship to familiar forms of activity — or means of expending them — can be measured by modern scientific means.

'Mark you, an absolute balancing of intake and energy output is next to impossible; but you need not bother much on that score for, as we have seen, the reserve will cover any slight deficiency which may arise while, should there be an excess of food, those bellows will work harder and cause the furnace to burn up a little more, which will be thrown off in heat. But if, year after year, you are eating more food than is required to meet the energy-demands you make upon your store, you will gradually tire the bellows working for you. More and more fat will be stored. You will have become an obesity "case"!

Reduce Slowly

'If that is your condition now, just think how it has been produced. Probably it has taken years for you to accumulate that excess of fat which is vexing you now.

'Do not expect to get down to a normal weight for your height and years in ten days; be distrustful of men or methods which offer to do it for you. Therein lies danger.

'In most cases it would be comparatively easy to any means the same thing as curing obesity.

'You do not want to be a human concertina — in for a short time, then out again! The restoration of that balance we have discussed, plus the repair of any damage which has been done, may take some time. But surely it is worth it in the long run.

'It should be your concern, whether as a person of normal or obese weight, to have knowledge of the various food values, and in particular to know which are fat-forming. You must have some means of measuring the value of the food you eat so that you can maintain a perfect balance of intake and output. But how?

Calorie Values

'It would be out of the question to take all foods and

FEEDING THE HUMAN FURNACE   45

beverages and show what activities each represents, so we have to rely upon a unit of measurement which works in this sphere much as a pound or a dollar does in money matters. A calorie measures food values just as litres or pints measure quantity; thus, by finding out the calorific value of the various foodstuffs, we can easily work out diets which are suited to our specific requirements.

'A calorie (more correctly a kilocalorie) is the amount of energy supplied by food-intake sufficient to raise a kilogram one degree Centigrade (1.8 degrees Fahrenheit) — which no doubt sounds highly technical! But the calorie does serve as a useful unit of measurement by means of which we cannot only calculate food values, but, what is more important, express the necessary requirements of the individual.

'How important it is that we should be able to use some such unit of measurement will be gathered from the fact that a kilo of shelled almonds equals nearly thirty kilos of tomatoes.

'If we did not know the vast difference in the calorific values of these foods, we should certainly never think of valuing them in such proportions. The point is that the bulk and weight of a meal simply does not matter.

'The meals that are primarily responsible for increasing your weight are those composed of calories derived from the fat-forming foods.'

Just what are the constituents of food that supply calories? They are carbohydrates, fats, proteins and alcohol. Carbohydrates can be regarded as complex such as starches, or simple like sugars. No matter which form they occur in, however, carbohydrates can be regarded as supplying 3.75 calories per gram or about 107 calories per ounce.

All proteins supply calories, from whatever their source, and the amount provided is 4.00 calories per gram or about 114 calories per ounce. It surprises many people to discover that the calorific value of protein is slightly higher than that of carbohydrate but the real difference lies in the proportion of each type of food constituent in the diet. Far more carbohydrate is eaten so it is this that contributes a large part of the calorie intake.

The largest calorie intake per gram is provided by fats. Whether of animal or vegetable origin (as oils), whether saturated or polyunsaturated, the fact remains that each gram provides 9.00 calories, each ounce 256. Unfortunately, fat also represents a growing proportion of our diet so the calories from it present us with a considerable portion of our calorific intake.

Alcohol has a calorific value of 7 calories per gram or about 200 per ounce, a figure almost twice that of carbohydrates. This means that a double measure of spirits contributes a staggering 250 calories.

Fats: 'Naturally, you will have to watch the fat-producing foods very carefully because they are the greatest contributor of calories. Any taken in excess of requirement will contribute to the formation of body fat.

'If, by the time you reach the dessert at dinner, you have already consumed a sufficient quantity of food to meet your energy requirements for the day, you will most likely complete the meal by adding some 300 calories which represent sheer surplus, or an increase of 28g (1 ounce) in body-weight.

'Much of the same result is achieved by the

person who obtains enough to meet normal energy requirements from actual meals, but who in the course of the day enjoys some ice cream, nuts, and sweets.

'People who say that they have eaten next to nothing have, very often, partaken of fat-forming foods such as these, failing to realize that, though the actual bulk or quantity may be small, the fattening power is big.

'It is usually the regular addition of such small amounts of surplus, as we have mentioned above, which account for fat folk in middle or late middle age.

'Add on your odd grams or ounces in this way for ten or fifteen years, and you will secure an accumulation which will not be banished in a few days or weeks, even if you suffer the starvation methods which find so much favour in some quarters — with almost invariable damage to health . . .

'You might suppose, at first thought, that a person who consumed a very considerable quantity of high calorific value must be intensely energetic, always full of vigour, and capable of getting through much more work than other people.

'It is in fact the case that when they are taken in excess of the body's requirements, they cause fat-storage in the body, with the result that, so far from being energetic, the individual concerned soon shows a tendency to tire quickly, and becomes lethargic.

'Apart from the performance of those tasks which we all have to perform, according to the nature of our work, recreations, and so on, the body's own daily routine makes its demands.

'In addition to the energy needed to carry on the work of the muscles used whenever we walk, run, talk, or make any movement, there is a continuous transformation of energy proceeding all the time.

'All the processes upon which life depends — the heart-beat, breathing, food-digestion — mean energy-expenditure. Thus, even while we sleep calories are being consumed.'

There is no need to cut out fat altogether. Remember that fat satisfies the appetite more completely than any other food. As long as the carbohydrate intake is left low it is possible that a moderate fat intake may cause weight reduction to occur at a greater rate than if the same number of calories are taken in other forms.

Practical experience has shown that most people who maintain a low carbohydrate intake can eat all the fat they wish and still lose weight. For example, individuals are less likely to eat more butter than their body really needs if they don't have much bread to put it on. A helping of fresh fruit with a little cream is less harmful in weight terms than tinned fruit with its accompanying high calorie syrup.

It is relatively easy to control the intake of visible fats like butter, margarine and cream, but the real danger lies in the foods containing hidden fats. High protein food sources like lean meat and cheese also contain fat — usually weight for weight with protein. Convenience foods are notoriously rich in fat and the increasingly popular fast foods often have high fat contents by their very nature. Similarly, pastry of all kinds, biscuits, sausages, pies, sausage rolls and the like, all contain high fat levels because it is impossible to make them without it.

Sugar: For overweight people, sugar must be regarded as one of the great enemies. Sugar sweetens but does not satisfy. In those with a tendency to put on excessive weight, who are already eating enough for their body needs, any sugar over and above this will turn straight into fat. Not only do sugary foods fail to satisfy hunger anyway, but in some people they can lead to a state of addiction, the so-called 'sweet tooth'. As sugar intake increases it is more rapidly and efficiently removed from the blood, leading in turn to a low blood-sugar. This mechanism is controlled by the hormone insulin. Too much sugar stimulates the production of too much insulin which, by lowering blood-sugar, creates the need to eat more. A low blood-sugar, called hypoglycaemia leads to dizziness, lack of concentration, irritability, and, what is of most danger to the overweight, it also causes the feeling of hunger. The answer is low-sugar, low-carbohydrate meals.

In attempting to lose weight, therefore, it is not sufficient simply to cut out sugar itself. The liking for sweet things must be reduced or cut out altogether. Artificial sweeteners like saccharin may help to reduce the calorie intake by cutting out sugar but they are not the answer. Replacing a calorie-sweetener with a non-calorie one does not reduce the desire for sweet things. The whole appetite for sweetness in foods must be curtailed. Saccharin is not put in cakes, sweet, biscuits, jellies and puddings yet they all supply sugar. What is required is the will to reduce the desire and intake of all sweet foods by training oneself to eventually dislike sweetness. It may take weeks or months to accomplish but once achieved, the reduced desire for sweet things is maintained permanently.

Once the desire for sugar has been overcome, it is then much easier to resist the temptation to eat sweets, chocolates, cakes, biscuits, jam, honey, syrup, tinned fruit, sweetened pudding and sweetened fruit drinks. Once this hurdle is passed, the road to permanently successful weight reduction is much smoother.

Starch: Bread, potatoes, rice, oats and cereal products are the main forms of high calorie starchy foods eaten in this country. Starch is composed of many units of sugar combined together so, after digestion, all starchy foods eventually end up as sugar. However, starch has recently been found to behave rather differently in the body than sugar. The reasons are mainly unknown but one factor may be that, because starch has to be digested first in order to be absorbed into the body, it takes longer to become assimilated. This means that starch in foods is less likely to put on weight than is pure sugar.

Nevertheless, the combination of bread and butter (or margarine) is fattening and for this reason the amount in any diet is restricted. Plain breakfast cereals, consisting of one type of grain that has been pre-treated in some way, and bran products are usually taken in helpings containing only a small amount of calories because of the bulkiness of the cereal as marketed. The average helping of cereals is less than 30g (1 ounce) and so provides only about 100 calories.

Starchy foods such as porridge, rice, macaroni, spaghetti, sago and tapioca tend to take up large quantities of water whilst being cooked so that the end product is bulky, but in calorific value the average helping may contain less than 100 calories. Porridge oats are particularly noted for a high uptake of water, some eight times their weight, so a helping of porridge is bulky, satisfying and low in calories.

Small quantities of these starchy foods can, therefore, be taken by most people on a long-term diet. They also provide dietary fibre which is a carbohydrate that is not digested. This has zero calories and is essential for supplying bulk to a food and so helping the digestive and eliminating processes. Although these cooked cereals are low in calories, their benefit as weight reducers is lost if they are swamped in sugar and cream. Learn to eat them as they are — any true porridge is flavoured with a little no-calorie salt.

Not everyone advocates low fat diets combined with high intakes of starchy foods, however. There is a book written by Dr Richard Mackarness, entitled *Eat Fat and Grow Slim* (Fontana, 1976). This work contains a foreword by Sir Heneage Ogilvie Consultant Surgeon, Guy's Hospital, London, and an introduction by Dr Franklin Bicknell, co-author with Dr Prescott of *The Vitamins in Medicine*.

Dr Mackarness points out that there are two types of people, viz: those who maintain a fairly constant weight throughout their lives, and those who fatten easily.

The cause of overweight, in his view (and it is supported by an impressive amount of scientific evidence) is that the obese are unable properly to 'burn up' the starchy and sugary foods they eat. This failure is thought to be due to a block in the chain of chemical reactions, consequent upon certain hormones and enzymes which they lack, or which their bodies may be unable to manufacture.

It is considered that they may fail to oxidize pyruvic acid properly, so that starchy and sugary foods, instead of being utilized to supply bodily energy, are deposited as layers of fat.

If a fat person stops eating starchy and sugary foods, he produces little pyruvic acid and thereby removes the bodily stimulus to make fat. Contrary to general belief, Dr Mackarness shows that fat is the least fattening of all foods, because it helps the fat person 'to mobilize his stored fat, as well as helping him to burn up the food he eats, more efficiently.'

He also claims that it is excess starchy and sugary food, not calories as such, that makes a person fat. Dr Mackarness deals trenchantly with what he calls the 'calorie fallacy' and explains that a calorie is a unit of heat, not a unit of nutrition. He advises the obese to forget about calories and to eliminate starchy and sugary foods from their diet, if they would reduce their weight to normal.

Fat people, he states, should also avoid beer and sweet wines, but may drink moderately of dry wines and spirits. Sugary fruits such as bananas, figs, dates, raisins, etc., should of course be eliminated from their diet.

Dr Mackarness advocates fat people eating to the limit of their appetites so long as they choose proteins, i.e., meat, fish, poultry, eggs, bacon, ham and cheese, together with such fatty foods as butter, meat fat, creams, milk and peanut butter. Unsaturated fatty acids (lecithin) are also recommended, especially for those with hypertension and heart disorders.

There is no restriction on fruits, other than the sugary fruits already mentioned, or on vegetables (except such starchy foods as potatoes, and sweet vegetables, i.e., beetroot, parsnips, sweet potatoes, and yams).

Dr Mackarness explains that by adopting the special diet he recommends, the weight of the obese person will not fall below that normal for their height and build, neither will it do any harm if they only want to lose a few pounds.

Sugar and Starch are the Culprits

He concludes his book by saying 'Starch and sugar are the culprits. Cut them right down and eat fat and protein in the palatable proportions of one to three. You will then grow slim while you eat as much as you like, and feel well because you will be eating the best kind of food. It is as simple as that.'

How much weight should you lose on the diet advocated by Dr Mackarness? If carried out faithfully, he claims that you can expect to lose as much as from seven to twelve pounds a month, and there will be no need, either, to go hungry or to count your calories in the process.

It should be pointed out, however, that this diet is not suitable for those suffering from gall-bladder failure or for sick people generally. It is intended only for those who fatten easily.

Proteins. The high protein foods consist of meat, fish, eggs, cheese, milk and fermented milk like yogurt. Excellent vegetable sources of protein include wholegrain cereals, peas, beans, lentils and pulses, nuts and root vegetables. Proteins are essential for repairing the effects of wear and tear on body tissues, so a certain minimum amount is required daily on any form of slimming diet. Proteins do not turn to fat as easily as carbohydrates do so that in most dietary regimes a moderate or large intake of protein is beneficial.

The advantage of protein is that it is satisfying as a foodstuff and it does not create an artificial appetite as do sweet things. Eskimos, who lived almost entirely on fat meat, only became overweight when they were introduced to sugar and flour. A diet based mainly on three large helpings of meat daily together with small amounts of fruit was started in the U.S.A. some twenty years ago and it is still popular as a weight-reducing diet in that country, where many people enjoy a high meat diet and can also afford to buy it.

The All-Protein Diets

The essentiality of protein in a daily diet has led to a concept in weight control where this foodstuff represents the sole source of calories. For short periods, usually for no longer than five days at a time, the individual eats pure protein, vitamins and minerals with adequate quantities of fluids. Over this period no carbohydrate or fat is eaten so that the body is forced to burn up its glycogen (liver starch) and fat stores in the production of energy for its daily functions. Hence the chance of weight loss is maximized. The diet has been advocated in the book *The Last Chance Diet* by Dr Robert Limm (Bantam Books).

To understand this concept it is essential to review the basic facts on the problem of overweight. The body requires only so much energy to function each day — there is the basic amount necessary for essential life processes plus a variable amount that depends upon the activity of the individual. Food intake is energy intake and if more energy is eaten than is used up, obviously the excess is stored and preserved as fat. Fat is stored energy. If the energy intake is consistently more than the energy output fat is deposited steadily and the individual gains weight.

These considerations apply only to those who have ceased to grow. During the growing period of a young person energy is required for growth and development and so metabolic requirements are difficult. Theoretically, therefore the simplest way to lose weight is to take in no food at all — in other words, to fast. With no calories coming in and a certain number being needed for life's processes and activity, the body must turn to its own stores of energy, namely glycogen and fat, and it must utilize these to provide the essential calories.

A fasting regime is not a good idea, however, because the body does not just restrict its energy source to unwanted fat. What happens is that it turns not only to fat stores for fuel but also to lean body mass such as kidney, muscle, liver and heart. Hence, energy is being produced at the expense of body protein and this is highly undesirable.

In fact, it has been estimated that, over the first month of fasting, half the body weight loss comes from lean body tissue. When body protein mass is burned up in this way it leads, on completion of the fast, to excessive eating to rebuild lost muscle and puts the faster into a 'negative nitrogen balance', a highly undesirable condition where nitrogen loss exceeds nitrogen intake. This problem is overcome in the total protein diet. As a total fast, no solid food is eaten but, to stop the body from using its own protein as an energy source and thus creating the 'negative nitrogen balance', the daily intake of essential protein is eaten without the accompanying fat and carbohydrate of an ordinary diet. As long as protein is being provided, loss of body protein is minimal at only 5% of any weight loss. The remaining 95% of any weight loss is provided by fat which is exactly what is being aimed at. The body stays in nitrogen balance and, since the lean body tissue has initially not been used up at all, there is no need for its replacement once normal eating is resumed. All that has been lost in providing energy is fat, and this is what every slimmer wants.

The minimum protein intake to be aimed at in such a diet is 45 grams daily. Hence in a three meal per day basis, each meal should provide 15 grams. As no carbohydrate and no fat is eaten, the calorie intake is only 60 calories per meal or 180 calories per day.

The usual procedure is to dissolve the protein powder in unsweetened fruit juice or vegetable juice, since these juices supply the mineral potassium which must be taken in any diet. Hence the 600 ml (1 pint) or so of these juices necessary to dissolve the protein themselves supply about 300 calories per day. A total daily intake of about 500 calories which supplies all the protein requirements must therefore represent the lowest energy intake conducive to health. At this level weight must be lost, since the deficit of 2000 or so calories required as a minimum daily energy expenditure must come from the fat reserves of the body.

It is equally important on such a diet to ensure the minimum of daily requirements of vitamins and minerals. These are best taken as one of the many excellent multi-vitamin/multi-mineral preparations available, but because potassium requirements are rather higher than can be taken in tablet form, this mineral is best taken as unsweetened fruit juice or vegetable juices. These juices, of course, are also excellent sources of other minerals and of vitamins.

Some people should not go on this all-protein diet. If you are suffering from kidney or liver disease or if you are pregnant, this diet is not for you. However what is very important for all is that the all-protein diet should not be used for more than 5 days at a time. A break of at least 3 days on a sensible normal diet should be taken between each 5 day regime of total protein. A more sensible way is to use the protein as a meal replacement for one or more meals once the 5–day diet plan has ended. The weight loss by the 5–day protein plan can stay lost if, on the sixth day, only two meals of pure protein are taken and the third meal is taken as a sensible balanced intake of all types of food. Thus, replacing two meals with the protein powder is carried on for a further 5 days, at the end of which only one meal is replaced by pure protein and the other two meals are sensibly balanced. This regime may be continued indefinitely.

'Name' meals do not mean vast intakes of food containing large amounts of calories. Sensible meals contain high protein sources such as lean meat, chicken or soya substitute, low starch and sugar intakes with plenty of vegetables and salads. Some carbohydrate must be eaten, but this is preferably in the form of wholegrains, wholemeal bread, mueslis and the like. These foods also supply essential dietary fibre to prevent constipation — one of the more common side-effects of slimming regimes. In this way, any weight lost during the initial 5 days on pure protein will stay lost and a steadier weight loss, obviously less dramatic than in the first 5 days, will continue while one or two meals daily are replaced by the powdered protein. It is also sensible to continue with vitamins and mineral supplementation whilst on any sort of meal replacement regime.

5

Food Values and Fundamentals

The Danger Foods
The foods, and other factors, responsible for obesity are as follows:

1. Eating more food than we need for our daily work. The body stores the excess in the form of tissue. The more we have stored, the less energy we are capable of expending. Our excess fatty tissue becomes an unsightly, burdensome handicap in all our physical and mental activities.

2. Eating far too much starchy food:
   bread — and butter   pies
   potatoes — and butter (or milk)   pastry
   porridge — and milk

3. Eating far too many sugary foods and drinks:
   sweet desserts   syrup
   ice-cream   honey

sweets   malt
chocolates   dates
bananas   figs
prunes   raisins
'colas' and other soft drinks, cordials, and squashes

4. Eating far too much fat-forming food:
fat meat cuts   rich desserts
fried foods   cream
cream cakes   butter

5. The eating of dead, devitaminized foods:
white bread   tinned foods
processed breakfast foods   white sugar
pickled and preserved foods sausage meats, etc.

6. A diet which consists largely of proteins and starches is the most common cause of constipation and glandular sluggishness. When the endocrine glands don't function normally, the body doesn't burn up its fuel so efficiently, and an unhealthy overweight condition results.

7. Lack of exercise. Most people after forty take no systematic exercise. Due to their devitalized diet, they scarcely have the energy for their routine duties of office or home. Even the will becomes affected by the daily diet, which is generally excessive in quantity and deficient in quality, i.e., deficient in the vital organic minerals and vitamins.

Watching Your Food Intake

Obviously, the first step in solving the problem of

excess weight is to pay attention to items 1 to 7 on the previous pages. This will involve some serious alterations in the daily diet.

Cut Out These Foods Altogether

The following foods must be cut right out if you would lose weight and gain health:

fat cuts of	white bread*
beef, mutton,	breakfast flakes*
pork and veal	cream
bacon	ice cream
fat ham	cream cheese
poultry (legs)	tinned milk (full cream)
salmon	powdered milk (full cream)
herring	margarine, dripping
whitebait	biscuits*
sardines	cakes
liver	condiments*
sausage meats*	jam*
sausages*	treacle
potatoes	golden syrup*
walnuts	white sugar*
peanuts	brown sugar*
peanut butter	almonds

The foregoing foods are either fat-forming, or are artificial aids to an artificial appetite. Those marked with an asterisk(*) are dead, devitialized foods and should form no part of the diet of any person seeking health. They are destroyers of health and the sooner people strike them off the daily menu the better.

All condiments such as pickles, sauces, chutneys, mustard, pepper, salt, etc., should be avoided because they stimulate the gastric juices and tempt one to eat more food than is necessary.

Foods to Be Eaten Sparingly
The foods and drinks to be taken sparingly are as follows:

Meats of all kinds. The average man and woman, not doing heavy physical work, should not have more than 170g (6 ounces) a day. People who are reducing require 225g (8 ounces) of protein daily.
Wholemeal bread — two or three slices a day are enough.
Butter — No more than 30g (1 ounce) per day.
Milk — No more than .25 litre (½ pint) a day.
Eggs — Two eggs as a change from meat.
Cheese — A small serving with your salad.
Beer, wine, spirits — All alcoholic beverages are stimulants to artificial appetite and should be reduced to mere token indulgence.

What You CAN Eat
After reading the list of banned foods and those of which you are counselled to eat sparingly you may well wonder what is left to keep you from starvation! Don't worry, there is plenty — and the best food in the world.

But certain new tastes may have to be cultivated, and this may take an effort of will. Without an effort of will, of course, you will never conquer the growing problem of excessive weight.

So better to start now while there is yet time to save yourself from becoming hopelessly entombed in flesh for 'the term of your natural life'.

After all, in the diet we are about to propose, you

are not asked to go hungry, or dispense with any really important food of first-class food value. You are not asked to become a food crank, a calorie crank, or renounce the pleasures of the table.

All that you are asked to do is to follow the advice of some of the world's greatest authorities on the subject of weight control and so order your diet that you will lose surplus weight and gain first-class health.

Fundamentals of a Health-giving Diet

We are all creatures of habit. And those habits can be good or bad, health building or health destroying — the choice is ours.

These habits can be altered or modified with a remarkably small amount of perseverance.

At the back of this book we set out a suggested daily menu.

Within the broad principles we have laid down in this book, this menu can be altered and varied almost without limit, depending upon the seasons and availability of foods.

There are certain fundamental principles of a healthy diet that cannot be ignored if we would bring our weight back to something like normal and raise the level of our health above normal. These principles are as follows:

Acid-Alkaline Balance

Man consists of many chemical substances, eighty per cent of which are alkaline and twenty per cent of which are acid-forming.

The proper chemical balance for health, therefore, and for keeping weight at our normal level (which is usually the weight we scaled at the age of

30) is maintained when our daily diet consists of this balance.

The foods which maintain the alkalinity of the blood are:
fruits
vegetables
salad vegetables
dried fruits

The acid-forming foods are:

meat	white bread
eggs	porridge meals
fish	rice
cheese	refined breakfast foods
sugar	spaghetti
tea	macaroni
condiments	coffee
biscuits	jams
pastry	nuts

New Knowledge of Food Values

The average overweight person will realize from the foregoing that, instead of eating eighty per cent each day of the alkaline group and twenty per cent of the acid-forming group, his diet for many years has been the other way round.

It has consisted of about eighty per cent of the acid-forming foods and only about twenty per cent of the first group. This, in brief, is the cause of his excess weight, his constipation, his sluggish, tired condition, with the threat of illness and disease making their first symptoms felt.

The time has arrived to make a change. It's a pleasant change, and from a health point of view, highly profitable. The second fundamental principle is equally important.

The old, indeed, the prevailing idea of food values, is that the food is rated highest which has the most solid texture.

By this theory meat, eggs, fish, cheese, bread, potatoes, etc., have that highest food value and fruits and salad vegetables have little or no value (as food) at all — pleasant in hot weather and all that, but no good to do a day's work on.

The Truth About Food Values

Now the foregoing attitude to these foods is a dangerous half-truth. It is precisely this popular misconception of food values which is responsible for the generally very poor health of the people of this country.

Let us get the facts about food rightly stated. The 'solid' foods (meat, eggs, cheese, fish, bread and potatoes, etc.) are of first importance, especially when one is engaged upon hard physical work, but even in these circumstances they should only form twenty per cent of our daily food intake.

The other eighty per cent should be made up of fruits, green leafed vegetables, carrots, beetroot, and milk. These are the vital foods, supplying the body with minerals, trace elements and vitamins.

The fact that these vital elements are generally under-supplied is the chief cause of the sickness and ill-health which is an affront to our intelligence in this country.

With persons of overweight, however, there needs to be some small modification of the foregoing. Milk must be limited to no more than half a pint daily or dried skim milk substituted for a full cream milk.

Other Considerations in Dieting

Fluids: The maximum amount of fluid drunk during the day is unimportant as far as permanent weight loss is concerned. What is important is that a certain minimum quantity of fluid is required, since water represents the main means of ridding the body of unwanted waste matter. There is no doubt that weight can certainly be lost rapidly for a short time by a reduction of fluid intake but it is not the long-term answer. A large part of the body consists of fluids and as water is relatively heavy it is very easy to lose a few pounds by denying oneself drinks or by sweating it out. Boxers use such methods in order to make a particular weight but they are not suitable for permanent weight loss. Once normal fluid intake is resumed the weight goes up again. Permanent weight loss can only be achieved by breaking down the body's stores of fat.

In women, the amount of water in the body is partly controlled by the female sex hormones which vary in blood concentration throughout the menstrual cycle. This is why many women put on several pounds in weight just before menstruation and promptly lose it when the menstrual flow starts. Doctors sometimes prescribe directions to help the woman lose this excess body water and such drugs, whether synthetic or of herbal origin, are often taken to help lose weight. Although effective in this respect, this loss in weight is only temporary so that diuretics will have no long-term effect upon the body weight.

Carbohydrates tend to cause retention of fluids and a large carbohydrate meal taken by a person who is trying to lose weight and breaks the rules even once can cause an apparent increase in weight of two or three pounds. This can be depressing unless it is realized that a temporary increase in weight of this sort is usually due to retained water, and the body soon rids itself of it.

Salt Intake: It is sometimes believed that eating less salt will cause less retention of fluid and so keep the weight down. This is true up to a point but, in the long term, salt intake is unimportant when long term weight loss is being considered. If salt is not eaten the equilibrium of the body is upset, just as it can be if too much is eaten, intake should be a happy medium. Salt is an acquired taste in most people, and the body does not need the excessive amounts eaten by many. It is also highly likely that too much salt taken regularly will lead later to blood pressure problems. The sensible rule for any slimmer is to take just the salt naturally present in food, plus a little in cooking, but add none at the table.

Frequency of Eating

Most people lose more weight if they eat three, four or even five small meals during the day than if they eat the same amount of food in one or two meals. This is because exercise taken after a meal increases heat loss from the body and therefore increases weight loss. If the metabolic rate is increased in this way four or five times a day more weight loss will occur than if it is increased only once or twice daily.

Some people starve themselves all day and then lose control of their appetite in the evening by eating a huge meal, containing a large amount of carbohydrate, not followed by any exercise. They would be better off having a substantial breakfast followed by other small meals during the day. However, dieting is very much an individual affair and some people can lose weight without much difficulty by controlling their appetite during the day whilst still enjoying a moderate-sized meal in the evening.

Problems for Those Trying to Lose Weight

Snacks: The most easily available snacks are, unfortunately, those which are the most fattening. Biscuits, bread and butter, cakes, sweets and chocolate are readily available in most households, and are most tempting. As an alternative, fruits of all kinds, with the exception of bananas, should replace these fattening snacks, when an individual is trying to lose weight. Those who get really hungry before they have time to prepare a substantial meal will find that hard-boiled eggs, cold lean meat, pickled herring, cheese and tomatoes, are satisfying alternatives.

Hunger between meals: There is no doubt that on any weight-reducing regime the main problem is hunger between meals. This can be overcome to some extent by taking materials in tablet or capsule form that swell in the stomach, when taken with a glass of water, and so relieve the pangs of hunger. The best swelling agents are those based on natural vegetable gums, such as guar gum. These gums have a dual effect. First, they supply bulk without calories, so giving a feeling of fullness. Secondly, because they are not digested, these gums act like any natural dietary fibre and, in the same way, prevent constipation. Although this is not a problem with those dieters who take note of the foods to eat and the advice given in this book, constipation is often a feature due to the decreased intake of food, when reducing weight.

Vegetable gums help prevent constipation without adding calories, and they are more efficient when taken with vitamins. Fortunately, the better preparations of guar gum also provide vitamins. Carboxymethlycellulose, and similar synthetic derivatives, should be avoided as swelling agents, as their safety has not yet been established in long-term use.

Drinks: Social drinking is always a problem for those trying to lose weight. A glass of beer or a single tot of spirits is roughly equal to 25g (1 ounce) of bread in calorific value. Bottled beers have slightly more food value than draught beer, and sweet cider, sweet sherry, port and sweet wines all have a higher calorie content than their 'dry' counterparts.

Sweet drinks should be avoided, not only because they are higher in calories but also as part of a general principle of avoiding sweet-tasting items of food and drink. It must be remembered, too, that the calorie content of drinks is increased by the addition of mineral waters and other mixers. Squashes, when diluted, contain slightly less calories than beer but, with the advent of low calorie mixer drinks and squashes, it is now possible to have thirst-quenching drinks without the calories.

Exercise machines: Machines such as stationary

bicycles and rowing machines, which enable people to exercise on the spot, can be useful for those who are unable to get enough exercise through sport or walking. The vibratory type of machine, where the subject is inactive, is of no value as far as weight reducing is concerned. In other words, it is not possible to massage weight away. In fact, more weight will be lost by casually strolling around than by using the machine for a similar length of time. What vibratory machines and manual massage do is to tone up the muscles, but they will not reduce the fat.

Spot reducers: It is not possible to lose weight exactly where you want to. No amount of localized massage, vibration or sweating under extra garments will break down the fat globules that you wish to dispose of. Sweating under specialized garments will cause a weight loss, but this will be regained immediately a drink is taken, so the weight loss will be purely temporary.

Usually, once a dietary regime starts to benefit you, fat tends to be lost from the places where it was last put on. This can lead to the minor tragedy of the middle-aged or elderly woman who finds that, on losing weight, her face loses its rounded contours before her bust, her abdomen or her thighs.

6

Vitamin and Mineral Needs When Reducing Weight

It has been estimated that some forty per cent of people in the UK are overweight. From the number of slimming regimes available and the advice given by experts (and others), it is obvious that removal of this excess weight constantly occupies the thoughts of many people. Here we are talking about overweight due to overeating. We are not concerned with white fat, brown fat, slow burners, fast burners or any of the other hypothetical concepts put forward to explain why some individuals are overweight. Nor do we consider excessive weight due to hormonal upsets or other medical problems or medical treatment, all of which are best left to the practitioner. We shall discuss, first, why people who eat too much are overweight and then consider the hazards that many encounter when embarking upon diets that are eaten with the prime purpose of reducing calorie intake but with little attention to the requirements of those other essential nutrients, vitamins and minerals.

The body requires only so much energy to function effectively each day, represented by a basic amount necessary for essential life processes plus a variable amount that depends upon the physical activity of the individual. Even the basic requirements vary amongst people and depend upon age, sex, height, body weight, mental activity and temperament. Basic requirements decrease with age after 25 or so years and it is the fact these are less but food intake remains unaltered that contributes to middle age spread. Food intake is energy intake because all food is capable of being converted into energy. When food that is eaten is not being converted into energy, it is stored within the body to be used at some later date. The storage of energy within the body is achieved in the main by the laying down of fat. Some is stored as animal starch or glycogen, particularly in the liver and muscles, but this should be regarded as the first-line reserves and is of no consequence in producing a condition of overweight.

Fat storage, of course, has other functions. It serves to act as an insulator against the cold and it is deposited around essential internal organs, such as the kidney, where it acts as a protective barrier. Fat is also nature's way of saving energy 'for a rainy day'. The conservation of energy as fat is of prime importance to wild animals, who eat when they can and have no guarantee of regular meals. They are able to live off their fat reserves until the next feed which can be hours or, more likely, days away. Most human beings have no such problems. Their three meals a day are virtually guaranteed and too often food intake is geared to appetite rather than to necessity. Small wonder then, that energy intake

VITAMIN AND MINERAL NEEDS

exceeds energy output with the result that the difference is laid down as body fat. We are laying down reserves of energy with little chance of ever using them. Body weight must increase under these circumstances.

It is important to realize that the three food constituents — carbohydrate, fat and protein — can all be converted by the body into fat. Many diets use the high protein concept where carbohydrate and fat intake are curtailed but lots of protein is eaten. This is fine up to a point but it must be remembered that gram for gram protein supplies 4.00 calories compared to 3.75 calories for carbohydrate. Excess protein is just as liable to be laid down in the form of fat as are starch and sugars. Fat of course contributes the highest energy at 9 calories per gram but don't forget alcohol at 7 calories per gram. Hence the ideal diet is balanced in these three basic food constituents but if this intake is reduced, other problems are introduced which are concerned with those essential food constituents, vitamins and minerals.

First we should consider why vitamins and minerals are so essential to life. The process of life depends upon thousands of chemical reactions that are going on in every living creature, plant or animal, every second of every day. These chemical transformations are called enzymes.

Enzymes are required to digest the food we eat, to convert that food to energy, to utilize that energy in muscles and to repair the body from the wear and tear that is produced by everyday living and increased by disease. Enzymes are the bases of life itself. In order to function effectively, however, enzymes in turn require other substances to be present, and these are the vitamins and minerals. When they are deficient enzyme efficiency drops and body processes slow down, then eventually stop. It is not difficult, therefore, to see how essential vitamins and minerals are in sustaining life. The body can make the enzymes it requires from the food. It cannot make vitamins and minerals so these must be supplied in the diet.

Foods vary tremendously in their content of vitamins and minerals, which is why only a balanced, good quality and varied diet will supply all the essential nutrients for health. Most vitamins are sensitive chemical compounds, which means that excess cooking or bad storage of foods can often destroy them completely. Minerals cannot be destroyed, but they are liable to be irreversibly bound to other food constituents making them unavailable to the body. Minerals in our food must ultimately come from the soil yet it is known that this varies widely in its mineral content and is often lacking in essential trace elements. Hopefully, though, a normal intake of food, taken from a wide variety of sources and cooked expertly, will supply all the necessary vitamins and minerals. How, then, can someone on a slimming diet with a restricted food intake hope to obtain their full requirements of these nutrients? The answer is that they are unlikely to. In fact, slimmers are now officially recognized as a group of the population who may be liable to vitamin and mineral deficiency when their slimming regimes are undertaken without professional advice.

Just how deficient in vitamins and minerals could an individual on a slimming diet be? If we take an average calorie requirement from a normal diet for

VITAMIN AND MINERAL NEEDS

an adult female to be, say, 2300 Calories and for an adult male 2900 Calories, we can assume that the amount of food supplying this would also supply the daily requirements of vitamins and minerals. When these people reduce their intake of food energy to the conventional 1000 Calories there must be a concomitant decrease in their intake of the essential nutrients. Unfortunately, however, the body's requirements for vitamins and minerals are the same regardless of the calorie intake. The only exception to this is thiamine or vitamin B_1 whose requirements are related to carbohydrate intake; the more carbohydrate eaten the more vitamin B_1 is needed. All other vitamins are necessary to health in minimum quantities that have no relationship to energy intake.

Individual items of food have varying contents of the various vitamins and minerals and, in avoiding some high calorie foods when on a slimming diet, there is a greater risk of deficiency in particular vitamins and minerals. Potatoes, for example, are our main source of vitamin C, not because they are the richest source of the vitamin but essentially because of the large bulk eaten. Unfortunately, potatoes are usually the first item of food that a slimmer will remove from the diet since they are also an excellent source of calories. The slimmer should therefore look to low calorie alternatives rich in vitamin C such as unsweetened natural fruit juices, raw fruit and lightly cooked green vegetables.

Cereals are rich in the vitamin B complex, yet slimmers tend to avoid these because of their high carbohydrate content. Bread is an important source of the vitamin B group and, as another example of a food usually taken in large quantity, it contributes a large proportion of these vitamins to the body.

Where, then, are the slimmers, who usually cut down bread, going to obtain their B vitamins? Most meats and particularly liver are very rich in the B vitamins so this presents no problem to the meat eater. However, the vegetarian can look to a variety of foods. Fortunately, whole raw nuts are a rich source of all these vitamins (apart from vitamin B_{12}) and remember that each gram will contribute a good share of the daily protein requirements. Eggs, of course, are a complete food that should feature in any slimmer's diet. Dried fruit will also yield useful amounts of the B group without making too large a hole in the calorie count. Green vegetables are good sources also but it is important not to destroy the vitamins by over-cooking.

It is unlikely that these vegetable foods will give you sufficient vitamin B_{12} and it is essential to ensure some intake of meats or dairy products on a slimming diet to ensure adequate amounts of this vitamin. The liver carries useful stores of vitamin B_{12} in most individuals, but on any long-term slimming regime these could be depleted if the intake of meat and dairy products is curtailed. Most dairy products are avoided by slimmers because of their high fat content, so it is important to make sure of one's vitamin B_{12} requirements by taking some meat.

Vegetarians may wish to obtain their B_{12} from low-fat cheeses at the expense of their calorie intake, but a supplement is the safest and easiest way to ensure their B_{12} requirements, and is, of course, essential for vegetarians at all times. Folic acid is unlikely to present a problem to the slimmer as the richest sources are green leaf vegetables and salads — both are foods that tend to be eaten in large quantity on a calorie-restricted diet. Liver, which is also useful in a slimmer's diet, is high in folic acid and has the advantage of being rich in the type of folic acid that can be used by man.

The vitamins most at risk in slimmers are the fat soluble A, D and E. This is because, by their very nature, they are associated with the fats and oils that the slimmers tends to avoid. During the winter months food is the important source of vitamin D, which is found in dairy products, fish and liver. A low intake of these will reflect in low body levels of the vitamin. In the absence of dairy products then a daily supplement is advisable. There should, however, be no problem in the summer as long as sufficient sunlight is allowed to fall on the skin, since the action of ultra-violet rays actually produce vitamin D in the skin.

The meat eater should derive ample vitamin A from liver as long as this is taken as part of the diet. Fish is also an excellent source of both vitamins A and D. The vegetarian will, hopefully, obtain his or her vitamin A from carotenes that are found in plants, but remember that not all carotenes will produce the vitamin. Carrots, spinach, broccoli and Brussels sprouts are particularly rich in carotene.

Vitamin E occurs in the highest concentration in vegetable oils and, although the slimmer may be wary of these in view of their high calorie content, some should feature in every diet. In addition, these oils supply the essential polyunsaturated fatty acids that are needed in many body functions. A daily intake of oils will therefore ensure adequate vitamin E and vitamin F (another name for polyunsaturated fatty acids). Vitamin E is widely distributed in many foods but its concentration is low and when the actual quantity of food consumed is reduced, as in the slimmer, a low intake of vitamin E follows. The simplest way to take vitamin E is capsules that contribute not only the vitamin but also the polyunsaturated fatty acids. The calorific value of these capsules is so low as to be negligible.

Meat and fish are generally regarded as suitable for slimmers and fortunately these foods are good sources of many of the vitamins mentioned. However, for a variety of reasons, such foods are not always eaten by the slimmer in sufficient quantity to yield the full complement of vitamins necessary. In addition, meat and fish are usually low in vitamins C and E, both of which are required in the highest quantities amongst the vitamins. Therefore a balanced diet should be sought, to incorporate other foods rich in these vitamins. Even so, on a daily intake of 1000 calories, there is the possibility of mild deficiency. Vegetarian slimmers are most likely to obtain a balanced vitamin intake but this is tempered by a lower bulk of food than is usual and their total intake is likely to be less.

The simplest insurance for anyone undergoing a slimming regime is a daily supplement of all the vitamins necessary to sustain life. We know that vitamins are essential in the processes of burning food to give energy, in the interconversion of foods and in the laying down of fat. Remember that these same vitamins are necessary to burn off that unsightly fat that is the aim of every slimmer. A deficiency of vitamins must reflect in a less efficient system for disposing of excess weight.

Minerals are just as important as vitamins to

VITAMIN AND MINERAL NEEDS

health and they act together with vitamins in controlling the metabolism of the body. We rely upon food as a source of minerals so that these too may be prone to deficiency as the amount of food eaten is reduced during slimming bouts. The minerals required in relatively large amount such as calcium and phosphorus are present in high concentration in dairy products but these foods are often ignored by the slimmer. Shellfish contribute reasonable amounts of calcium and phosphorus but they are not acceptable to the vegetarian. Bread and cereals are a good source of calcium but these, too, are foods generally avoided by slimmers. Vegetables must therefore be the most important source of calcium and phosphorus to the slimmer. Our skeleton acts as a rich reservoir of calcium but, during prolonged periods of slimming, the withdrawal of calcium and phosphorus from bone could tend to weaken it. In the absence of dairy products, then, a supplement of calcium must be sought.

Magnesium is widely distributed in all foods but the reduction of calories to 1000 or so per day must adversely affect the intake of this mineral. Low magnesium in the body leads to irritability, depression, mild mental problems and muscular weakness. How often are these conditions associated with the slimmer! Magnesium is best taken as a supplement in the form of dolomite tablets. These supply calcium as well and the two minerals are in the same ratio in dolomite as in the required intake from food. They are calorie-free and dissolve in stomach acid to ensure good absorption.

Even on normal diets supplying the average calorie requirement, iron is often at risk because of its poor absorption. The possibility of deficiency must therefore increase on a reduced calorie intake. Again, the meat eater has some advantage over his or her vegetarian counterpart because the iron from meat is better absorbed than that from vegetables. Under normal circumstances this does not matter, because the vegetarian makes up in quantity of vegetable foods what they lack in quality, but a reduction in food intake will almost certainly give rise to iron deficiency. In the female of childbearing age this deficiency may be exacerbated by menstrual loss of iron and the chances of full replacement on a slimming diet are remote. Therefore, the slimmer must choose foods with a high iron content — usually of animal origin — but failing this they should seek a supplement.

Iron from iron salts is notoriously difficult to absorb so that the quantity of salts taken are far in excess of that needed. Iron amino acid chelates are the nearest equivalent to the iron presented in meats (although of vegetable origin) with the result that absorption is superior to that of iron salts.

Zinc is another mineral assuming more and more importance as research continues, and it tends to be associated with high protein foods. Hence any slimming diet that is low in protein-rich constituents will be deficient in zinc.

There is considerable doubt as to whether conventional diets provide sufficient zinc, so the chances of deficiency from a calorie-reduced diet are enhanced. Seafoods are particularly rich in zinc and they contribute other minerals from the sea as well as protein, at the expense of a few calories. Nuts are also good sources of zinc so that the non-fish eater can obtain some of their requirements from these.

VITAMIN AND MINERAL NEEDS

The simplest way to ensure a good intake of trace minerals daily, particularly whilst slimming, is to take kelp. Kelp is dried seaweed that has, concentrated in it, all of the minerals of the sea, probably the richest source of minerals anywhere in the world. In addition, kelp is an excellent source of iodine which has a very important role in the body. Iodine is a constituent of thyroxine, the hormone from the thyroid gland that controls body metabolism. Low iodine levels mean a sluggish metabolism which is the last condition a slimmer would want. By ensuring an adequate iodine intake, a slimmer can make certain that the body has every chance to metabolize its food, and more importantly that excess fat, into energy. In addition the other, minerals in kelp are essential ingredients in the enzymes necessary for the metabolic conversion of food and fat into energy.

There is little doubt that people will continue to undertake slimming diets without medical supervision for a long time to come. As long as they are aware of the need for (1) a minimum intake of calories (2) a minimum intake of protein and (3) a supplemental intake of all vitamins and minerals, they should come to no harm. At least it is possible to ensure an adequate supply of vitamins and minerals using supplements that yield only a negligible quantity of calories. Supplementation removes some of the problems associated with dieting. All that is left then is an awareness of protein intake and the pleasures of calorie-counting.

7

The Experts' Views

A Harley Street Specialist's Views
Dr Eustace Chesser, a Harley Street specialist on weight reduction, writes in his book, *Slimming for the Million*:

'Nobody gives us our fat. We add it to ourselves. The implements we use for the purpose are the knife, fork and spoon; the materials, the fat-forming foods.

'I fully realize that forbidden fruit is apt to taste sweeter than any other! Nothing arouses desire more strongly in many people than that a thing should be banned, whether it be a book, a play, a course of conduct — or an article of diet.

'Yet the fact remains that right through life we are constantly having to exercise self-control for worthwhile ends. Whenever we take a step forward we have to leave something behind — often something we like.

'However much we may enjoy the fattening

morsels (or more-than-morsels!) we cannot hope to succeed in reducing excess weight if we are unwilling to give up, for our health's sake, those fuel foods from which fat comes — the fats, carbohydrates and alcohol.

'No half measures will suffice, and no compromise of the "just this once" order should be tolerated. We need never rise from the table feeling hungry; we need not go thirsty; but we must stop consuming the foods and beverages which form fat.

To Get Rid of Fat, Stop Eating It!

'Fat people often have thin memories — they forget that the weight they want to drop took years to acquire. A week or two of careful avoidance of the fattening foods, is followed by a return to them. They are like a magnet on some people.

'Clearly, determination is needed if you are to resist the appeal of rich, fat-forming foods, but there is always some means by which you may strengthen your effort, and that is by reminding yourself of your aim. Whenever you feel tempted to slip back to the old, bad diet habits, call to mind two points:

1. That you add fat to your body by eating it;
2. That your ideal or normal weight is linked with better health and appearance, whereas obesity means discomfort, ill-health, and unshapeliness.

'This use of your aim will help you more than anything else to avoid slipping back, and in time you will find that your taste is tending to change; for our food preferences are largely due to habit.

'Every week you abstain from fattening foods you not only keep the enemy away, but strengthen your own power to continue. Each day the effort grows less.

Be Honest With Yourself

'You must be honest with yourself. Either you avoid the fat-forming foods and lose weight, or you continue to take them, and add weight. It is easy to find excuses for eating the things you like.

'But the fat man who stoutly maintains that he thrives on fat, never felt better in his life, and so on, may deceive his friends, and even himself — but never his doctor. 'The obese woman who scoffs at efforts to reduce as being merely a foolish fashionable whim or something dangerous, is simply justifying her weakness.

'One's friends too, are apt to be the opposite of helpful.

'It is not so much those who sneer at efforts at weight-reduction — they are merely ignorant, and you can afford to ignore them.

'Far more dangerous are the solicitous friends or relatives who mourn your loss of weight and insist that it cannot possibly be good for your health.

'"Why," they say, "you used to look so fit and strong; now you're becoming a mere shadow of your old self!" It never occurs to them, and no amount of explanation or reasoning can convince them, that fat is a burden, a disability, and the firm friend of many other ills.

'While you are fat, you are well; loss of weight must mean ill-health, as they see it. They mean well, and it is very hard to go against their wishes, especially if, as is often the case, they are of one's own family. But well-meaning ignorance is just as dangerous as any other kind.

'You must, if you are to make any progress at all in your efforts to reduce, stop consuming fattening foods; if you are unwilling to make the effort involved, there is no point in reading this book. Its whole purpose is to outline a treatment, in which rigid reduction of the fattening foods is the first essential, and which has been amply proved by my professional experience to be effective.

Calorie Values Compared

'Here it is worth examining the values of the substances which are found in the different foods, most of which contain two, and some three, of the following:

Protein – fuel value of 28g (1 ounce) = 123 calories.
Fat – fuel value of 28g (1 ounce) = 279 calories
Carbohydrates – fuel value of 28g (1 ounce) = 123 calories.
Alcohol – fuel value of 28g (1 ounce) = 210 calories.

'Note the high calorie value of fat; it is clear that foods in which the proportion of fat is high will, if given a prominent place in any diet, soon result in more fuel than is needed by the human furnace. But the other substances listed are also fuel-providers.

'So we come back to our starting point, and find that if we are to fix responsibility for excess weight, the fat man or fat woman is the guilty party — through eating fat-forming foods. Rich foods are fat foods; fat folks usually love them! They demand cream, butter, olive and vegetable oils, fat meat, milk with cream in it, pastries made with lard and butter, and all kinds of dishes which have been cooked in fat . . .

'Remember that carbohydrates enable fat to be stored which, in the ordinary way, would have been burned up in energy. Thus carbohydrates cannot only be judged by their calorie value.

'It is not only the obese who need to avoid the fat-forming foods. Those who, after treatment, have found their weight restored to normal can only hope to keep it thus by holding the fattening foods at arm's length.

'Patient and physician alike always need to bear in mind the basic truth that fat comes from food, and food only; it comes not from water, nor from the heavens, and the sooner that simple truth is recognized, the better.

'Prolonged excess of food intake over energy output nearly always leads to overweight.

'But this is by no means all. In time, the metabolic processes become affected. There is interference with the weight-regulating mechanism, the glandular system, and other organs of the body . . .

Obesity's 'Bad Brothers'

'When obesity invades the organism, even though its progress may be slow and, at first, almost invisible, slight ailments almost invariably accompany it. They may be so slight, indeed, that the patient and even the physician may fail to detect them.

'They are obesity's "Bad Brothers" — or some of them. For if the condition is not corrected, other unpleasant relations of obesity will probably come, either on a short visit or to stay.

'Long lists of ailments which are produced or complicated by obesity are often published in books on obesity and, indeed, it is easy to make an impressive catalogue which shows how vital it is that obesity should be regarded seriously.

'I shall not attempt it, for it is unnecessary. What matters is that the patient, and his physician, should both clearly appreciate that there is no disease which is not aggravated by obesity, no operation which is not made more difficult by it, no condition in which its burden is not real and oppressive.

'Quite apart from the proneness of the obese to such ills as diabetes, gallstones, circulatory failure, and other complaints, the overweight patient cannot put up so good a fight, and his chances of recovery are lessened, in any illness. Pneumonia provides an outstanding example of this; obesity tips the scale against recovery.

'Aesthetic considerations count for much, as any obese patient will admit. Alteration of the shape, always in the direction of the unshapely; reduced skin vitality, so that its softness is lost.

'If at first it seems difficult to change dietary habits, it is necessary to bear in mind one important point — that appetite is very largely a matter of habit, both as regards the quantity and the nature of the foods required.

'The stomach is as big as its contents. If you have grown accustomed to heavy meals, then the stomach will seem to expect them, for it has become fitted to take a large quantity.

'Actually, however, its size can vary from next-to-nothing to the volume of the largest meal you can consume, and if each day you are in the habit of eating large meals, and suddenly change over to small meals, the stomach will protest.

'This may show itself in the form of nausea, faintness, if not severe indigestion. There is no necessity for this. The bulk of the meal can, and should, be made up of the non-fattening foods. The capacity of the stomach depends upon the quantity eaten.

'As regards the nature of the foods, this again is largely a matter of habit. Many men who thought they never could drink tea without sugar managed to do so, and like it after a time, when during war-time they served in areas where sugar was not available for months on end.

'You can develop a fondness for many foods by regularity in taking them.'

Dr Gayelord Hauser's Views

Dr Gayelord Hauser is perhaps the most eminent of the American nutritionists. Many Hollywood film stars, who dare not put on weight or get ill (without jeopardizing their huge salaries) are under Dr Hauser's personal supervision. His advanced dietetic principles have achieved remarkable results, and his patients swear by him.

In his book *Diet Does It!*, Dr Hauser has a very valuable contribution to make to the problem of losing weight and gaining health.

In a chapter entitled 'Solving the Reducing Problem for a Lifetime', Dr Hauser writes:

'The smaller your waistline, the longer your lifeline, so life insurance companies show us by actual statistics.

'The smaller-waisted people are the ones privileged to enjoy longer lives, not those with lots of avoirdupois in the middle.

'Just as an artist moulds his statues from clay and bronze, so we can mould and re-mould our bodies with delicious but non-fattening foods. Any person alive, provided his bone structure is normal, can have a trim, vital body if he is willing to work for it.

'During this reducing regime, you can build up your health until you have more energy and are slimmer and trimmer than you have been in years.

'Now let us face facts. If you are overweight, you have eaten more foods than your body needs, and the excess has been stored as fat.

'This statement remains true regardless of how little you eat in comparison to a slender, active person . . .

'This principal reason overweight people fail to reduce is their wrong approach. For example, many of you tell your friends that you are overweight because of your glands.

'You know perfectly well, and so do your friends, that this remark is only an alibi.

'Probably only one per cent of the people who have made themselves believe that they are fat because of glandular disturbance actually have anything wrong with their glands.

'In any case, glandular health can be helped by a correct diet, especially iodine and the B vitamins, and by the removal of excess weight.

'Your alibi is hollow. Do not use it, for every time you do, your friends put their tongues in their cheeks.

Health versus Food
'Many people are overweight because they are bored, troubled, or emotionally upset. They gorge

themselves as an escape mechanism in the same way that an alcoholic drinks to forget his difficulties.

'They go on candy drunks, carbohydrate drunks, and dessert drunks.

'When they have their minds on eating they are not thinking of their problems. Such people do not realize they are eating for this reason, and they are often the first to condemn the alcoholic as lacking character. When their true situation is brought into the open, the correction is easy.

'Other people are fat because they over-emphasize both the pleasure of eating and the hardship of denial.

'Their sense of values is faulty, and they are actually saying that the pleasure of eating is greater than good health and looks.

'What they fail to realise is that they can learn to enjoy eating non-fattening foods just as much as fattening ones, provided they set out to develop tastes for the right foods.

'The person who strictly avoids cake, coffee with both cream and sugar, and other fattening foods, can quickly come to dislike them.

A Sound Reducing Diet is a Healthy Diet
'Some fat people will tell you that they have inherited their tendency to be fat. I say they have also inherited their cook books. Many people fail to reduce because they have tried a few times, failed, have become discouraged or perhaps ill, and have decided they cannot reduce. They rationalize that staying fat is the best policy.

'Great strides have been made in scientific reducing in the past years until it is now possible to build and improve health while you are reducing; in fact, a well-planned reducing diet is one of the most healthy diets you can eat.

'You can have plenty of food and need not be hungry, but the wallpaper-paste foods, such as white bread, refined cereals, cakes, cookies, and pastries of all varieties, which can in no way build health, must be avoided.

'Thousands of people stay on low calorie diets all their lives and are aware of it; they do it not from choice but because they enjoy non-fattening foods more than fattening ones.

'If your reducing is to be successful, you must join their ranks. These are the people who do not like sweets and desserts.

'It is not the occasional holiday dinner that puts on the pounds. It is certain types of food which you eat day after day, such as bread with every meal, too many desserts or too much candy, or cream and sugar in coffee.

'Unless you are willing to change your habits of eating, do not bother to reduce, for, regardless of how many pounds you lose, you will gain them back as soon as you again eat an excess of high calorie foods.

'You can develop a taste for any food provided you eat only a little of it at first, increase the amount as you come to enjoy it, and eat the same food time and time again.

'Every food you now enjoy you have cultivated a taste for in exactly this manner. Learning to enjoy non-fattening foods is far more important than the number of pounds you lose, for when you have actually acquired a taste for low calorie foods your weight problem is solved for a lifetime.

'Eating vital foods rich in vitamins and minerals can help you to normalize your appetite.

How to Make Reducing Easy

'Our first concern, therefore must be in choosing foods which will made reducing easy for you and, at the same time, will build up your health.

'Make sure that your protein intake is high; proteins help to keep the body firm and prevent extra wrinkles, so have one or two eggs daily and, if available, a serving of lean meat.

'These may be prepared any way except fried. A good serving of cottage cheese may be used as a meat substitute or in place of the eggs.

'Most of the proteins of vegetable origin, such as nuts, beans, peas, and lentils, are high in calories; therefore the protein need must be met largely with fat-free proteins of animal origin.

'Aside from foods that supply proteins, vegetables and vegetable juices should make up the greater part of the reducing regime. Choose green or yellow vegetables most frequently. These vegetables have a high vitamin and mineral content which is essential to build your health, and their bulk helps to prevent hunger.

'Raw vegetables digest much less completely than do cooked vegetables; hence they should be used most generously. The following vegetables may be eaten in any quantity desired.

'Vegetables in the column on the left contain three per cent sugar, those on the right, five per cent sugar:

asparagus	beets
Brussels sprouts	cabbage
celery	carrots
cucumber	cauliflower
leeks	onions
lettuce	pumpkin

spinach
squash
vegetable juices made
  of above

radishes
string beans
tomatoes
turnips
vegetable juices
  made of above

'Lima (broad) beans, peas, corn, potatoes, sweet potatoes, and yams are about twenty per cent sugar and should be avoided if you seriously wish to reduce.

The Fruits that Can Be Eaten Freely

'Grapefruit, oranges, fresh loganberries, raspberries, strawberries, blackberries, fresh pineapple, raw, peaches, apples, apricots, grapes, etc., can be freely used.

'All canned fruits containing refined sugar supply, by weight fifteen per cent sugar, whereas bananas and fresh figs, plums, and prunes are more than twenty per cent sugar; therefore these should be avoided if you have many pounds to lose.

'Dried fruits, all of which contain at least seventy-five per cent natural sugar, should be strictly avoided.

'Either fresh or canned tomatoes or tomato juice are usually available and so universally enjoyed that they become an excellent source of vitamin C. Drink as much tomato juice as you like and have tomatoes daily either stewed or in salad, soups, and aspics.

'Fresh vegetable juices are excellent sources of vitamin C if drunk immediately after they are made; their vitamin content will depend on the vegetables from which they are prepared. A grapefruit and an orange may be eaten daily to supply this vitamin.

Importance of B Complex Vitamins

'The foods listed can supply all of your body needs except the vitamins of the B Family. These vitamins are so important during reducing that their value cannot be over-emphasized.

'If they are amply supplied, you can lose that constant craving for sweets which results when vitamin B_1 is so meagre that sugar cannot be used efficiently in your body.

'These vitamins help to give you vigour which will make you feel like exercising and hence help you to reduce faster.

'Best of all, these vitamins help to build and maintain the health of your skin, eyes and hair so that the longer you reduce the more attractive you become.

'Unfortunately the ordinary sources of the vitamins of the B Family (although actually poor sources) are high calorie foods: whole grain breads, cereals, and foods such as macaroni, noodles, and spaghetti made of whole grains, beans, peas, lentils, and nuts.

'Wheatgerm, having a much higher content of B vitamins than the foods already mentioned, can be used by people having only a few pounds to lose, but it varies from 100 to 300 calories per half cup, depending upon the variety used.

'The food which offers the most vitamins and the least calories — only 20 calories per heaped tablespoonful — is powdered brewer's yeast.

'For the first week of your reducing regime, take a tablespoonful of yeast stirred into water or tomato juice after each meal.

'This amount can then be reduced to a tablespoonful daily, but you will feel better, have more pep, nicer skin, and build greater health generally if you continue the three tablespoonfuls daily. Should the powdered yeast prove disagreeable to you mix it in fruit juice or try to take it in tablet form.

Weight Reduction Requires a Mental Effort

'If you are serious about wanting to build your health and at the same time to lose unsightly pounds, eat only the foods already discussed.

'Avoid all denatured breadstuffs, pastries, desserts, sweets, fats in all forms, nuts, gravies, and the high calorie vegetables and fruits.

'Realise that learning to enjoy low calorie foods — and you can learn to enjoy them only by eating them — is far more important than the number of pounds you lose.

'Think of your programme, not as a reducing diet, but as a regime which builds health and solves the weight problem for a lifetime.

'Your mind, you know, is like a radio dial, in that you can tune in any station you desire; you can feel sorry for yourself and let your thoughts dwell on chocolate creams you are denying yourself, and eventually fail; or you can have a feeling of superiority, knowing full well you are tackling your problem with wisdom and that you are solving it once and for all by learning to enjoy low calorie foods so much that you will want to continue eating them throughout your life. Again, an intelligent attitude determines your success or failure.

'Plan varied, interesting, attractive meals for yourself. Be especially careful to eat between meals.

'Your midmeals should be near enough to the next meal to take the edge off your appetite. The menus at the end of this book (pages 102–4) show you how appetising your meals can be.

Let Your Mirror Tell the Story
'Fresh carrot sticks, celery, or the juices taken between meals are important. These midmeal feedings prevent you from getting so hungry that you will want to overeat at meal time.

'They also increase your efficiency to such an extent that they should be continued throughout life.

'After you have lost as many kilos as you desire you can add to your diet more fruits, fruit juices, cheeses, and perhaps a slice or two of whole grain bread daily.

'In general however, you should continue to choose your foods, first to build health, and, second, for their low calorie content.

'The speed with which you reduce will depend entirely upon how closely you adhere to the regime. The longer you follow the reducing regime the more you enjoy low calorie foods and the less trouble you will have in keeping off any unwanted pounds during the years to come.

'A person who has only ten pounds to lose and takes it off in two weeks often does not learn to enjoy low calorie foods enough to eat them indefinitely; hence he regains them and must usually fight weight until he learns to enjoy the foods on a reducing diet.

'If you have fifty or more pounds to lose and feel it is impossible to reduce so much, set out to lose five pounds; when that is accomplished, set a goal of another five pounds, and continue in this manner until you reach your ideal weight.

'Start today and do not stop until your mirror

shows a reflection which pleases your eyes and your head is held high with pride of accomplishment. Keep this one thought always in your mind: diet does it — it is impossible to fail,' Dr Hauser concludes.

Weight Reduction Should Be a Slow Process
Dr W. F. Christie, in his book *Ideal Weight*, says: 'By a rapid loss we mean a reduction in weight of 3 to 6 lbs. in a week. Such a loss is detrimental if continued. The destruction of a large amount of fat may produce a surplus of fatty acids which circulate in the blood and poison the tissues (acidosis); muscular and heart weakness is apt to occur; the pangs of hunger may be a real punishment, conducing to irritability of temper, nerves on edge, attacks of faintness and dizziness, with hunger pains over the heart.

'By slow reduction, we mean a weekly loss of up to 1 kilo (1–2 pounds). It is a convenient and safe method which can be continued over long periods, provided that suitable subjects are chosen.

'A relatively large amount of meat eaten in a slow reduction diet may injure those whose kidneys are already impaired . . .

'The total extent of reduction must be a personal issue with each fat subject, the ideal stopping place being that at which one feels healthiest and happiest.

A Good Reduction Diet is Safe and Sure
Dr Christie continues: 'Having determined the calorie value of the maintenance diet, we are enabled to form a reducing diet on a scientific plan.

'In it the fuel foods are restricted to such an extent that fat is withdrawn from the reserve depots within the body in order to make good the deficit in the day's ration.

'Since 25g (1 ounce) of human fat is worth 279 calories of heat and energy, it follows that a consumption of food which is less than the maintenance diet by 558 calories will result in a daily loss of 50g (2 ounces) of body fat, or nearly 1/2 kilo (1 pound) a week in body weight. Simple multiplication of these figures will vary the loss proportionately.

'Because fat is laid down very slowly, its rapid removal must be unnatural. Wrinkling and bagginess of the skin are apt to occur as the tide of fat subsides, while some muscular and heart weakness is inevitable.

'The devotee of speed in the game of losing weight neither looks well nor feels so fit as the man who takes it off more slowly, of equal importance, perhaps, is the fact that he learns very little of the fat-forming qualities of the various articles of food, and is just as likely as formerly to put on weight after he has lost it.

Fitness and Weight Reduction Go Together

'A slowly reducing diet is carried out at home. It does not interfere with the pursuit of the day's business or pleasure. It gives quite enough to eat, especially if food is thoroughly masticated.

'Moreover, it is safe; those who follow it feel unusually fit throughout the period of dieting.

'Its effects, too, are likely to be permanent; because a considerable latitude in the choice of food is permitted, the reducer takes an interest in, and learns to avoid, those items which are particularly fat-forming. Very seldom do weights go up afterwards.

'Prolonged vigilance on the part of the reducer is essential for success. Unaccustomed feelings of well-being, greater freedom of movement and improvement in looks help to sustain interest.'

In regard to the diet, Dr Christie sounds a note of warning:

'It is necessary to include in every diet a certain amount of concentrated carbohydrates, like bread, toast, biscuits, rusks, breakfast cereals, potatoes, bananas, etc, to ensure that the body will burn its own fat properly.

'If it is not so included, acidosis will develop. Some of these foods should be taken at breakfast or afternoon tea. They may be chosen according to the patient's desires, he alone knowing which ones render the diet palatable to him.'

According to Dr W. F. Christie fatty deposits are formed very slowly and their hasty removal by unwise slimming processes is unnatural. A too-rapid burning up of fat weakens both heart and muscles, and is conducive to attacks of faintness and dizziness. Moreover, when weight is lost too rapidly, the skin cannot adapt itself to bodily changes and hangs in unsightly folds and wrinkles, making one look prematurely old. For these reasons, it is imprudent to seek to lose more than one pound per week.

Reducing Drugs Should be Shunned

Fortunes have been made by the sale of weight-reducing drugs, medicines and pills. Most of these are worthless, the rest are dangerous. Writing on this subject Dr Chesser said:

'Just consider, for instance, those advertisements for purgatives which appear year after year claiming that one has only to take small doses regularly in order to become slim and fit.

'If their claims were anything like true, the blot of obesity would long since have been erased in "England's green and pleasant land".

'But it is there still, though millions of pounds are poured into the pockets of manufacturers of these "remedies" each year. One preparation which had an enormous sale in Great Britain was analyzed by a chemist engaged by the British Medical Association.

'People had been eagerly buying it at an exhorbitant cost, but the analysis revealed that the contents of each bottle were worth only three per cent of its retail price.'

What of the Glands?

There is a good deal of misconception in regard to the part played by the glands in putting on surplus flesh.

When we see people who are so fat that they have become virtual freaks, there is no doubt that their endocrine glands have run amok.

But what caused this glandular abnormality in the first place? Chemical imbalance in the body. In short, a bloodstream devoid of the essential vitamins and minerals. Vitamins have been described by scientists as 'the food of the glands' — the activators of the body's organic functioning.

When the essential minerals — of which there are fifteen — and the vitamins — of which there are twenty or more — are seriously under-supplied, glandular and/or organic abnormalities arise. The stimulation of the endocrine glands usually gives rise to abnormal appetite, and fat formation follows as surely as night follows day.

To avoid the possibility of abnormal glandular functioning, see that you obtain the essential vitamins and organic minerals and adopt the diet which follows.

8

Weight Reducing Diet

The following diet may be varied to suit all seasons and tastes by using the calorie value lists on pages 105–9.

- *Before Breakfast*: Large glass of diluted orange and lemon juice (one orange, half a lemon) or one vitamin C 50mg tablet.

  Breakfast: Four teaspoonsful wheatgerm, with small quantity of milk or skim milk and stewed apricots.

  Mid-Morning: Tea and wholemeal bread and butter — one slice bread. Gradually cut out sugar in tea.

  Lunch: Large green leaf salad with lean ham. Fruit dessert.

  Afternoon: Tea and wheatmeal biscuit with yeast extract spread.

  Dinner: Grill (no fat) and vegetables (no potatoes). Fruit dessert.

  Before retiring: One teaspoonful of molasses,

followed by a cup of tea or fruit juice.

●*Before Breakfast*: Iced tomato juice (tinned brands are recommended).
Breakfast: Wheatgerm and milk or fruit juice. Two or three diced peaches.
Mid-Morning: One slice toast with little honey, and tea.
Lunch: Two lean cutlets and pineapple. Apples, peaches or pears for dessert. (No bananas or 'sweet' fruits.)
Afternoon: Tea and wheatmeal biscuit.
Dinner: Large green leaf salad, including chopped parsley, grated apple and carrot, with a little grated cheese or hard-boiled egg. Fruit dessert.
Before retiring: Teaspoonful of yeast extract or molasses in hot water.

●*Before Breakfast*: One grapefruit.
Breakfast: Poached egg on toast. One slice toast with a 'scrape' of butter. Cup of coffee.
Mid-Morning: Tea and wheatmeal biscuit with yeast extract spread.
Lunch: Generous salad — lettuce, tomato, parsley, celery, cucumber, with lean cold roast beef. Fruit.
Afternoon: Tea and wheatmeal biscuit with a little honey or yeast extract spread.
Dinner: Grill or fish, and vegetables. Fruit.
Before retiring: Teaspoonful of molasses in lemon juice and hot water.

●*Before Breakfast*: Pineapple juice.
Breakfast: Grated apple, wheatgerm and milk.
Mid-Morning: Tea, wholemeal bread, butter and honey (one slice).

Lunch: Large salad and cold mutton or 50g (2 ounces) Cheddar cheese. Fruit.

Afternoon: Tea and wheatmeal biscuit with honey or yeast extract spread.

Dinner: Grilled fish and vegetables. Fruit in season.

Before retiring: Molasses and tea.

Calorie Consideration

The calorie used in food chemistry is the kilocalorie, not the small calorie, (used in physics).

Calories are units of heat and the kilocalorie represents the amount of heat required to raise the temperature of one kilogramme of water (approximately one quart) by one degree Centigrade (1.8 degrees Fahrenheit).

One hundred kilocalories will raise the temperature of a quart of water from 0 degrees Centigrade to 100 degrees Centigrade or from 32 degrees to 212 degrees Fahrenheit, which expresses a great deal of heat.

Calorie Value of Foods Per 100g (4 Ounce) Portion

SALAD VEGETABLES
(Low Calorie Foods)

	Calories
Celery	21
Cucumbers	20
Onions	48
Tomatoes	26
Cabbage	28
Asparagus	26
Radishes	26
Carrots	53
Lettuce	14
Watercress	36

RAW FRUITS
(*Low Calorie Foods*)

	Calories
Cantaloupe	29
Papaw	58
Watermelon	35
Grapefruit	50
Lemons	27
Oranges	50
Quince	20
Mangoes	92
Blackberries	68
Raspberries	57
Loganberries	64
Strawberries	45
Apricots	85
Nectarines	84
Peaches	47
Pears	48
Bananas	115
Pineapple	50
Cherries	91
Grapes	85
Plums	48
Prunes	69
Apples	72

COOKED VEGETABLES
(*Low Calorie Foods*)

	Calories
Beans (French)	23
Beetroot	48
Broccoli	34
Chard	28
Spinach	14
Carrots	36
Cauliflower	17
Kohlrabi	17
Onions	47
Parsnips	57
Pumpkin	38
Potatoes	113
Sweet potatoes	258
Tomatoes	26
Turnips	27
Cabbage	19
Celery	6
Peas	145

PROTEIN FOODS

	Calories
Beef, roast	185
Beef, steak	175
Ham	248
Mutton chop, lean	155
Lamb chop, lean	140
Eggs and bacon	380
Veal chop, lean	172
Veal cutlet	180
Liver	130
Pork, roast	205
Pork, chop	215
Sweetbreads	220
Chicken, broiled	156
Chicken, roast	210
Duck, roast	208
Turkey, roast	195
Goose, roast	335
Beans, baked	150
Beans, soy	170
Cottage cheese	141
Cheddar cheese	380
Egg (one)	80
Swiss cheese	420
Yogurt	60
Milk, cow's	85
Milk, goat's	112
Milk (skim)	47
Fish, average	140
Oysters, raw	57
Salmon (tinned)	240
Sardines in oil	385

HIGH CALORIE FOODS

For purposes of comparison, the following high calorie foods are listed

	Calories
Butter	960
Margarine	960
Jams	300
Doughnuts	500
Bread (white)	320
Biscuits (oatmeal)	514
Lard, refined	1120
Cornflakes	460
Honey	407
Chocolate creams	810
Milk chocolate	678
Ice Cream	240
Wholemeal	470
Raisins, seedless	410
Almonds	800
Brazil	860
Cashew	760
Peanuts	680
Peanut butter	750
Walnuts	874
Coconut, fresh	720
Sugar, white	480
Sugar, brown	420
Waffles with butter	530
Cream, double (heavy)	430
Cream, medium	372

Note: Nuts are classified as protein.

Vitamin Dosage

The following should be taken three times a day after meals. They can be taken all together:

- 1 Vit. B_1 (10mg) tablet
- 2 Vit. B Complex tablets
- 1 Vit. C (50 mg) tablet
- 1 kelp tablet

NOTE: *The B complex vitamins, Vitamin C and the iodine content of kelp, all assist in converting food into energy, and thus prevent it being stored as fat.*

Index

acid-alkaline balance, 63
    acid-forming foods, 64

body types, 25

calories, 44, 45, 85, 104, 105
carbohydrates, 40
Chesser, Dr Eustace, 24, 31, 42, 82-83
Christie, Dr W.F., 97-99

diets and dieting
    all-protein, 54-58
    health-giving, 63
    frequency of eating, 67
    help in reducing, 91-92
    safe dieting, 97
    reducing drugs, 99
    recommended diet, 102
Dobbs, Sir Charles, 39
drinking, 69
Dublin, Dr Louis I., 15-16

exercise, 20
    lack of, 34, 60

fats, 18-19, 46-48, 60, 72
Fisk, Dr Eugene, 23
fluids, 66
food
    values, 59, 64-65
    danger foods 59-61
    acid-forming, 64
    those maintaining alkalinity, 64
    vitamin and mineral content, 74
    calorific values of 107-109
food addiction, 33, 35-37
fruit, 93, 106

Hauser, Dr Gayelord, 88
heart disease, 14
heredity, 32
hunger, between meals, 68

insurance
    statistics on being overweight, 12, 15
    general standards, 23

Johnson, Dr Harry, 17-19

metabolic rate, 39

obesity, 24, 42
overweight
    the dangers of, 12
    in USA, 16
    in Great Britain, 16
    in Europe, 16
    in women, 21
    social factors, 35
    ailments associated with, 86-87

proteins
    all-protein diets, 54-58
    protein foods, 108

salt, intake, 67

starch, 50-51, 53, 54
sugar, 49, 53, 54

vegetables, calories in, 105, 107
vitamins, 71, 94, 110

weight
    ideals, set by insurance companies, 12
    reduction, 20-21
    in general, 26
    tables, 27-29
    gain, 31
    reasons for losing, 40
    reducing slowly, 44
    problems associated with loss, 68 ff
    reduction and mental effort, 95, 97
    reducing drugs, 99
    reducing diet, 102ff
women
    overweight in, 21
    social factors, 35